To Max and Grace, the lights of my life.

Guiding Yoga's Light

Lessons for Yoga Teachers

Nancy Gerstein

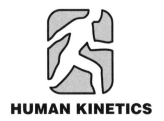

HUMAN KINETICS

Library of Congress Cataloging-in-Publication Data

Gerstein, Nancy, 1958-
    Guiding yoga's light : lessons for yoga teachers / Nancy Gerstein. --
Rev. ed.
        p. cm.
    Previous ed. published in 2004 by Pendragon Publishing.
    ISBN-13: 978-0-7360-7428-5 (soft cover)
    ISBN-10: 0-7360-7428-7 (soft cover)
    1. Hatha yoga--Study and teaching. I. Title.
    RA781.7.G44 2008
    613.7'04607--dc22

                                                    2008013940

ISBN-10: 0-7360-7428-7
ISBN-13: 978-0-7360-7428-5

This book is a revised edition of *Guiding Yoga's Light: Yoga Lessons for Yoga Teachers*, published in 2004 by Pendragon Publishing.

Acquisitions Editor: Gayle Kassing, PhD
Developmental Editor: Cynthia McEntire
Assistant Editor: Scott Hawkins
Copyeditor: Erich Shuler
Proofreader: Anne Myer Byler
Graphic Designers: Joe Buck, Fred Starbird
Graphic Artist: Francine Hamerski
Cover Designer: Keith Blomberg
Photographer (cover): Neil Bernstein
Photographer (interior): Neil Bernstein
Photo Office Assistant: Jason Allen
Art Manager: Kelly Hendren
Illustrator: Jen Gibas
Printer: Sheridan Books

Printed in the United States of America   10 9 8 7 6 5 4 3

The paper in this book is certified under a sustainable forestry program.

Human Kinetics
Web site: www.HumanKinetics.com

United States: Human Kinetics
P.O. Box 5076
Champaign, IL 61825-5076
800-747-4457
e-mail: humank@hkusa.com

Canada: Human Kinetics
475 Devonshire Road, Unit 100
Windsor, ON N8Y 2L5
800-465-7301 (in Canada only)
e-mail: info@hkcanada.com

Europe: Human Kinetics
107 Bradford Road
Stanningley
Leeds LS28 6AT, United Kingdom
+44 (0)113 255 5665
e-mail: hk@hkeurope.com

Australia: Human Kinetics
57A Price Avenue
Lower Mitcham, South Australia 5062
08 8372 0999
e-mail: info@hkaustralia.com

New Zealand: Human Kinetics
P.O. Box 80
Torrens Park, South Australia 5062
0800 222 062
e-mail: info@hknewzealand.com

Be a lamp to yourself.
Be your own confidence.
Hold on to the truth within yourself as to the only truth.

Buddha

Contents

Preface

Happiness comes when your work and words are of benefit to yourself and others.

—**Buddha**

The title of this text not only describes the guiding role of the yoga teacher, but also how the very essence of yoga practice guides and enlightens the student within his or her own existence. Students learn to incorporate the teachings into their daily lives, whether by learning to be patient with their children, by dealing with life's inevitable changes, or by simply breathing away anxiety. For the curious and introspective yoga teacher, serious yoga student, or fitness instructor who has a desire to step out of the bounds of asana teaching, *Guiding Yoga's Light* succinctly distills the principles of yoga's science and philosophy as it integrates them into the body, mind, and spirit.

In this expanded edition, we are pleased to offer three new, teacher-requested chapters: Salutations in Motion, Lessons of the Heart Center, and Relaxation Lessons. These new chapters enhance the text that became a highly sought-after yoga teacher's reference tool after its initial publication in September 2004.

Guiding Yoga's Light interprets yoga's 4,000-year-old philosophy in an effort to inspire, delight, and enable yoga students to go deeper, both in their physical practice and in their lives. Each lesson demonstrates to teachers and to their students how to readily bring the relevant and systematic teachings of yoga off their mats and into their lives. On a more universal scale, the book's message is that the strength, balance, and stretching of the physical practice work deeply into all aspects of our collective consciousness.

The lessons in this expanded version of *Guiding Yoga's Light* follow the same general six-step format as the original.

1. Intention. The introductory information sets up the meaning of the day's class and creates awareness of the particular yoga experience.

2. Approximate time. The length of each written lesson script is provided in order to help yoga teachers plan their classes. If you want to add to or edit the lesson, please note that any changes or added pauses will alter the approximate length of the script. The timing does not include the time required to teach asanas.

3. Lesson. The lesson is the core of the class, the essence for the day's teaching. The next three information blocks—asanas for deepening, practice off the mat, and wise words—grow from this core lesson as they help enhance and thread the class.

4. Asanas for deepening. The suggested practice illustrates through body stretch, movement, and sensation how to feel the lesson within the body. These asanas are suggestions only. Please be sure to include the asanas that work best for your teaching practice, style, and student level.

5. Practice off the mat. This practice may be used as a homework assignment, reminder, or topic for discussion to integrate the lesson within your students' daily lives.

6. Wise words. Quotes, quips, and other suggestions end each lesson. These proverbs are intended to engage your students within the context of the lesson.

This book is organized so that the beginning student or teacher can journey through the various aspects of yoga by first understanding the foundation of hatha practice. The lessons must first be learned in the body before they can spread throughout the mind. For instance, chapter 1 contains lessons that are important, if not crucial, for novice students—the basics of breathing and benefits of practice. Chapter 2 builds on that knowledge to include more specific breathing exercises beyond simple diaphragmatic breathing. Once the lessons in chapters 1 and 2 are processed, the student will be better prepared to understand the physical and spiritual philosophy of the postures and salutations presented in chapters 3 and 4. Accordingly, the lessons in the succeeding chapters open up to the subtleties and tactics of practicing and living the yogic lifestyle. This includes the explanation and classroom encounter of the yamas and niyamas, as well as the various lessons of relaxation, the heart center, chakras, emotions, and mindfulness. Presenting the lessons in this systematic manner suggests that yoga is a continuous new discovery that extends far beyond the boundaries of the printed word.

However, the experience is the best teacher of all.

Acknowledgments

This work would not be possible without the guidance of the thousands of yogis who came before me. I humbly thank Swami Rama for the teachings he has imparted most graciously through his books and lectures, as well as the gifted and generous teachers he trained. I'd also like to thank Sandra Anderson and Rolf Solvik, who are the real deal, the truest of yogis I have ever met. Thank you for sharing your scholarly wisdom of the Himalayan teachings.

Thank you to Kate Palandech, who published the original work.

A tremendous thank you and *namaste* to the incredible spirits I had the pleasure of working with at Human Kinetics: acquisitions editor Gayle Kassing, for your natural foresight and understanding about living the full yoga experience; developmental editor Cynthia McEntire, a guiding light in clarity, creativity, and organization; and Neil Bernstein for his masterful photography.

Thanks also to yoga teacher Howard Davis of Tenth Gate Yoga, who skillfully and joyfully modeled for the asana photographs.

I would like to acknowledge the blessings and energies of so many divine souls who helped me shine my light even during some fairly dark times. You have all been spiritual mentors extraordinaire and taught me that the prana that exists in love can move mountains. Thanks to Bobbie Rudman, Louie Gerstein, Judy Marcus, Don Gerstein, Allan Marcus, Judith Pownall Gerstein, Marcie Lance, Mindy Kagan-Bernath, Deb Salmon, Sharon Duberstein, Megan Tyner, and Laura Chernaik. I love you all.

I want to thank my very best teachers—my students. Please accept my gratitude. I am truly blessed to have the most wonderful job in the world: to look into your faces and experience the wonder and truth of yoga.

I thank the divine that I was chosen not only to discover the path of yoga but to write about it.

Finally to Max and Grace, who will always have the cutest little asanas I know.

Introduction

Your work is to discover your work and then, with all your heart, to give yourself to it.

—Buddha

What is this love affair we have with yoga? The practice itself is time-consuming and laborious, but it's also serendipitous and full of excitement. It's a wonderfully curious adventure, a momentous discovery, and a quiet trip into our inner world all rolled into one. Each instant on this yogic path holds the opportunity to feel spacious, connected, and so much more alive.

Since the beginning of my journey into yoga, I've cherished how the ancient teachings apply to every aspect of modern living. Be it our jobs, relationships, child rearing, errands, the grief of losing a loved one, or the challenges of riding life's ongoing crises, the lessons of yoga can be found everywhere. Perhaps this love affair with yoga is grounded in the eternal love of life itself.

Guiding Yoga's Light is a starting point, a tool for bringing the wealth of the yogic experience into the daily lives of both teachers and students. Over the years, I have recorded my various lesson plans in order to keep track of where I've been as a teacher and where the yogic path has taken me as a student. These lessons have proved to be a rewarding guide that motivates me on this journey and that helps me focus my intentions on my own practice.

It is not my objective to make all classes the same, but rather to offer a template to explore each yoga lesson wherever it may lead. Armed with the knowledge that our yogic ancestors have provided, I feel that we must seek to create an experience that is vital and current to modern students while keeping the traditional meanings intact. It is with great joy and love in my heart that I venture this text as a tiny step toward meeting that end.

TIPS FROM THE FRONT OF THE ROOM

Since you are offering your guidance of the yogic experience, it's imperative to continually work at balancing the various aspects of your own life. Be aware of how you live yoga philosophy, knowing that practice begins every time you take a conscious breath, movement, or thought. How you implement what you learn along the road will profoundly affect your teaching. The following recommendations will help you balance your class as well as your guidance:

- Have a relaxed presence. Until you feel calm, simultaneously take and teach the class. Do what feels best in the moment so that you can give and share the best of what you know. Remember, you are the guide; if you radiate light and love, your students will sense it.
- Enjoy the day's lesson. Discover what it means to you so that you can put your heart into it.
- Teach what you need to learn. You will be more passionate about your teaching and ultimately be a better teacher.
- On days when you feel that you have nothing to give, remember that just your physical presence, smile, and voice can be enough to make a difference to your students. Never underestimate the power of just being you.
- Take a lesson from the student. Don't compare yourself to others, including other teachers. Everyone has their own light and their reasons for living the yogic journey.
- Teaching is a joy and privilege. It is your path and your profession to help others find healing, space, and inner peace. Make every moment count.

EIGHT LIMBS OF RAJA YOGA

Raja means "royal." Raja yoga delineates the path of yoga in its highest, most comprehensive form.

Gathered by the sage Patanjali Maharishi in his *Yoga Sutras*, the eight limbs are a progressive series of disciplines that purify the body, mind, and spirit, leading the yogi to enlightenment and liberation from suffering.

First Limb: Yamas—Moral Disciplines and Restraints

Ahimsa—Nonharming, nonviolence

Satya—Truthfulness

Asteya—Nonstealing

Brahmacharya—Moderation in all things

Aparigraha—Nonpossessiveness

Second Limb: Niyamas—Observances

Saucha—Purity

Santosha—Contentment

Tapas—Determined effort

Svadhyaya—Self-study

Ishvara Pranidhana—Surrender to the divine

Third Limb: Asana

Posture

Fourth Limb: Pranayama

Regulation or control of prana

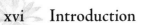

Fifth Limb: Pratyahara

Withdrawal of the senses

Sixth Limb: Dharana

Concentration

Seventh Limb: Dhyana

Meditation

Eighth Limb: Samadhi

Superconscious state

In many Western yoga classes, stepping onto the eight-limb path begins by learning the discipline of hatha, the physical yoga practices intended to eliminate distractions from the mind by first stilling the body. These practices exhibit that once the body's energies are freed and awakened, the student is more physically and mentally available to understand and implement the deeper aspects of the eight limbs: right and mindful living (including the yamas and niyamas), asana, pranayama, and finally, the internal steps that lead to meditation and samadhi.

The lessons outlined in *Guiding Yoga's Light* begin with the initial discovery of body and breath awareness, then gently prepare the student for the more advanced practices of yoga's science and philosophy. When we are ready to receive the teachings, a new world appears before us.

Namaste.

Your yoga begins when you leave the classroom.

It's how you connect to people and how you relate to the world.

Your yoga is the giving and receiving.

It's the wellness between inner and outer worlds.

Your yoga is living the purpose of your life.

Your yoga is to spread peace, one person at a time.

The light and love in me

bows to the light and love in you.

Om.

Shanti, shanti, shanti

Chapter 1
Beginning Lessons

Words have the power to both destroy and heal. When words are both true and kind, they can change our world.

—Buddha

During the first few weeks with your new class, you, the yogic guide, have much to teach your students.

For new yogis, the primary focus is on asana—postures—and on opening the outermost layer of our consciousness—the body. This opening, strengthening, and ultimate aligning of the body clear the nadis, the subtle energy channels of the body and enhances the flow of prana, or life force. Guided by mind and breath, the heightened flow of prana creates changes on physical, emotional, and spiritual levels. Most students feel the effects of practice their first time on the mat.

For experienced yogis, practice profoundly affects mental and spiritual layers by calming the mind and awakening intelligence throughout the body. We experience a deeper understanding of our essential nature and the world. The practice becomes a quintessential ingredient in living a more fulfilling, healthier, and awakened life.

Whether your class consists of new or experienced yogis, please consider the following points when structuring your lesson plans:

· Hatha yoga is not simply an exercise system. It's a 4,000-year-old holistic path of health and self-development that begins by using the body to influence all aspects of our being.

· Never underestimate breath awareness. The breath is the link between body and mind. Demonstrate and teach the practice during every class. Mindful breathing during class can make the difference between achieving the holistic effects of asana and simply stretching.

· Practice is both individualistic and systematic. Encourage students to challenge themselves to begin the process of change, but to back off the physical practice when they feel pain. This requires the practice of inner listening. Students should never force asana or breath. Accepting the body as it is in the present moment is integral to the practice.

- Keep a beginner's mind, an open mind. Remind students that every day on the yoga mat is new and different. As the Japanese Zen monk Suzuki said, "In the beginner's mind, there are many possibilities; in the expert's mind, there are few."
- Have fun with your lesson plans. Teach the lessons *you* want to learn. This ensures that your lessons come from the heart.

First Class Facts

Intention

To give beginning students a foundation of yoga and establish the intent for each week's class.

Approximate Length

3 to 4 minutes

Lesson

Hello, I'm [your name here] and welcome to the ancient science of yoga. Before we begin, I want to mention a few things to make your experience in yoga class the best it can be.

- Yoga is practiced in bare feet, so please take off your shoes and socks. Our feet have tiny receptors on the bottom; when our feet are bare, we can feel the earth beneath us. Practicing yoga in bare feet also helps improve our balance.
- Come to class on an empty stomach. Wait about two or three hours after a big meal, or about one hour after a snack.
- Please turn off your cell phones.
- Try to come to class a few minutes early. Consider being prompt a part of your practice.
- Let me know of any preexisting injury or special conditions so that I can help you. No matter what physical limitations you have, there are many ways to practice the postures.
- Do your best to let go of any competitive mind-set you may have. Yoga is absolutely noncompetitive. It's not just a workout; it's a spiritual practice that makes the body stronger, more flexible, and generally healthier. The aim is to calm the mind, open the heart, and stimulate your spiritual evolution.

Within the last few years, the practice of yoga has been praised for its stress-reducing properties. Basically, the process works like this: stress and tension cause the body to tighten up. Tension blocks energy flow. In yoga, we use asanas (postures) and breathing to open constricted areas of the body and mind. This helps to release and erase tension. As the body relaxes and opens, the mind becomes calm and less busy. When the mind is less busy, negative feelings such as anxiety, fear, and anger melt away. The mind begins to open up to positive feelings such as patience, acceptance, and compassion.

Practicing yoga is a process. It's not about getting poses picture-perfect. It's about being sensitive to your body and being quiet enough to hear your inner voice.

The one ground rule we have is to please stay within your physical limitations. This means listening carefully to what your body is telling you and honoring its messages, erring on the side of safety. If you want to grow and heal, you have to take responsibility for listening to yourself.

And most of all, have fun. This should feel good!

[It is recommended this script be followed with an introduction into diaphragmatic breathing. See the next lesson, page 6.]

Asanas for Deepening

These opening asanas allow beginning students to awaken their bodies through gentle and subtle methods. Since this may be their first lesson in body awareness, these postures—reclining twists, leg cradle, reclining hamstring stretch, and sitting on toes—concentrate on the most prominent points of beginning practice: opening the back and feeling the spine, feeling the feet on the earth, and stretching the breathing anatomy and other areas where breath is naturally blocked—the ribs, waist, and hips. These movements ultimately help the student feel and release the breath.

Reclining Twists

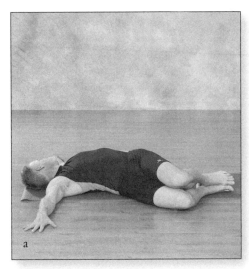

Knee over knee

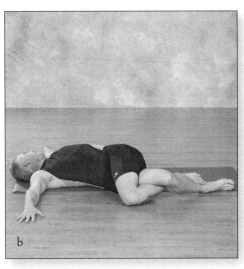

Eagle legs

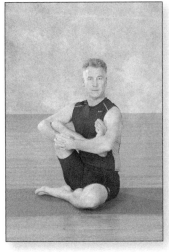

Leg cradle

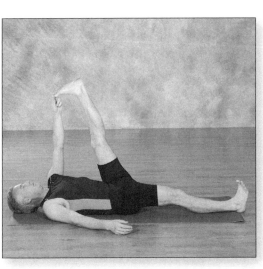

Reclining hamstring stretch

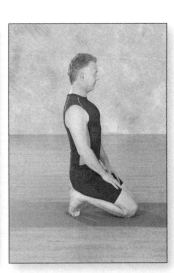

Sitting on toes

Practice Off the Mat

Keep your attention on what you're doing. When your mind wanders off to matters of the past or the future, factors such as work, worries, or responsibilities, bring it back to the moment.

Wise Words

Listen to your inner teacher. He or she has much to teach you.

Sensation is the language of the body. Listen to what the body is saying.

Yoga is a time-tested path for developing a deeper experience of yourself and the world.

Be kind and loving to yourself by accepting yourself as you are.

Many of us are physically stressed because we believe our minds and bodies are separate.

Learning Diaphragmatic Breathing

Intention

To illustrate and educate students on the value of diaphragmatic breathing.

Approximate Time

6 to 8 minutes

Lesson

The foundation of our yoga practice is learning to breathe properly and completely. This means breathing from the diaphragm, or diaphragmatic breathing. Diaphragmatic breathing allows us to slow down our heart rate, bring our blood pressure down, clear our minds, and relax our muscles. In fact, it's the most important thing we can do to reduce everyday stress. When we're not breathing fully, blood pressure goes up, heart rate increases, muscles become tense, and even our thinking becomes scattered.

Breathing properly is not just the foundation of yoga; it's the foundation of life itself. It's the first thing we do when we're born; it's the last thing we do when we die. You can live a few weeks without food, but only a few minutes without breathing!

So let's learn diaphragmatic breathing.

Begin in shavasana, feet about 12 inches (30 cm) apart, arms at your sides, palms up. Take a moment to dismiss any thoughts other than being here in this room. Sweep those thoughts out of this room. Leave your past and your future. Keep your attention here in the present moment. Don't let go. This is your time to look inward and to take care of your well-being. In doing so, you'll be better equipped to handle life's challenges.

Close your eyes and focus on your breath. As you breathe through your nose, bring all your awareness to your breathing. Notice if your breathing is shallow or noisy. Is your inhale the same length as your exhale?

Bring your focus to the space between your nostrils. Feel the coolness of the inhale, the warmth of the exhale. By focusing here, you're starting to turn inside.

The idea is to slide into an awareness of the breath—gently. No forcing. No pushing. Just remain present to the coming and going of breath. When the mind wanders off to work or to family or to responsibilities, simply bring it back to the breath. Back to the breath.

Now we'll make sure that we're breathing completely from the diaphragm. First, soften the belly. Consciously release any tension you may be holding there. Then put your right hand on your abdomen and put your left hand on your chest. If you are breathing diaphragmatically, your right hand will move up and down as your abdomen naturally extends out on the inhale and goes back down on the exhale. Your left hand should stay relatively still. [Pause long enough for students to take three to five breaths.] If only your left hand is moving, you are breathing from your chest, and you are getting only about one-third to one-half of the oxygen you would get from diaphragmatic breathing. [Pause and walk the room to observe the students.]

If you're not getting it today, keep trying. We'll breathe diaphragmatically through the nose throughout class. Breathing through a posture helps us relax through it.

The deeper you breathe, the more relaxed and focused you become. Never forget to breathe.

Every inhale brings in fresh prana, life force. Every exhale releases the toxins and tensions of the day.

Being sensitive to the whole body, we breathe in. Being sensitive to the whole body, we breathe out.

No striving, no forcing.

Asanas for Deepening

The reclining side stretch and sitting side stretch open the intercostal muscles between the ribs, aiding diaphragmatic breathing.

The clam is a simple forward bend from an easy pose.

As the student performs makarasana (crocodile), he or she should feel the breath fill the lower back.

During the uttanasana (standing forward bend), remind students to sense how the breath vibrates the torso.

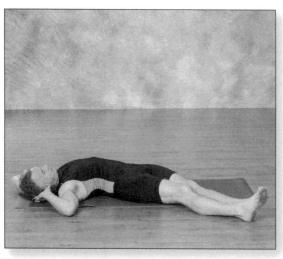
Reclining side stretch

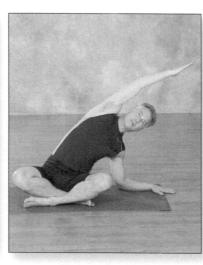
Sitting side stretch

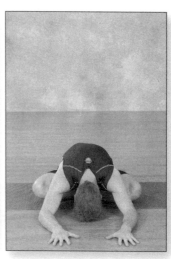
Clam

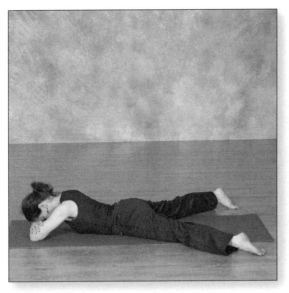

Makarasana

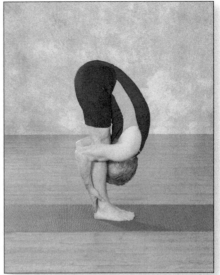

Uttanasana

Practice Off the Mat

Practice diaphragmatic breathing for five minutes a day either in shavasana or makarasana (crocodile). When you are able to use the diaphragmatic breath to keep your emotions in balance, you'll discover the value of breath awareness.

Wise Words

Gently nudge your tight areas with breath.

Diaphragmatic breathing is innate. Babies do it without any training. Later in life, when stress sneaks into our consciousness, we forget how to do it.

Yoga is preparation for living. It gives us a curiosity and enthusiasm to participate in life.

The breath is the link between mind and body.

Benefits of Yoga

Intention

To create awareness of the benefits of yoga practice.

Approximate Time

2 minutes

Lesson

Lie in shavasana, feet about 12 inches (30 cm) apart, arms at your sides, palms up. Rock your head from side to side until you find the flat part on your skull. Rest your head there.

Feel your abdomen rise and fall with each breath. Imagine your lungs as a pair of balloons, filling as you inhale and emptying as you exhale. As they fill, they become longer and rounder; they grow in all directions. You begin to feel the air going into the back, into the chest, sideways down the waist, every breath elongating the spine.

Yoga is a practical philosophy that involves every aspect of our being. It teaches us both self-discipline and self-awareness.

At the physical level, yoga gives us relief from many illnesses or diseases. The postures strengthen and stretch the body and create a feeling of well-being. Yoga sharpens the intellect and improves concentration. Our breathing practices calm the mind.

Spiritually, yoga introduces us to inner awareness and gives us the gift of stillness.

Yoga is a journey toward inner peace. Let's begin our journey.

Asanas for Deepening

During the cat stretch, become aware of the whole body, from the top of the head to the soles of the feet. Move with the breath, inhaling at the navel center (photo *a*) and sending it through the body as you exhale (photo *b*).

Many beginning students find that hip openers can uncover secret blocks of trapped energy that cause tension through the back and hamstrings. While practicing the reclining hip openers, focus on the physical and emotional edges of the stretch. Relax into the limitation and see if you can stay with the pose for one more breath. Notice what's stretching—is it your muscles or your patience?

Spinal rocks provide a lively way to soothe and awaken the spine. Roll several times, building momentum with the breath. Exhale up to a seated position (photo *a*), and inhale as you roll back (photo *b*). Feel the spine tingle.

Cat Stretch

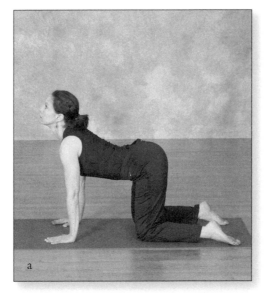

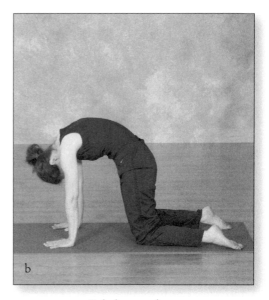

Inhale, release down

Exhale, stretch up

Reclining Hip Openers

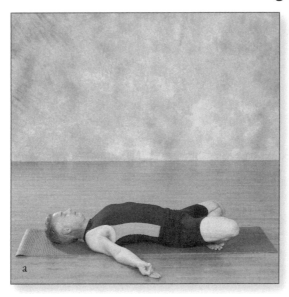

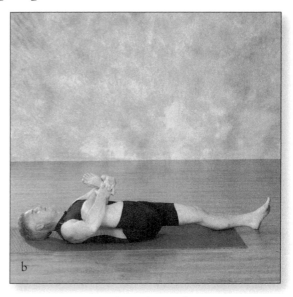

Reclining easy pose

Reclining leg cradle

Spinal Rocks

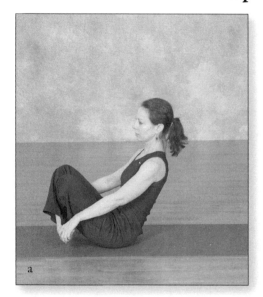

Exhale, sitting up

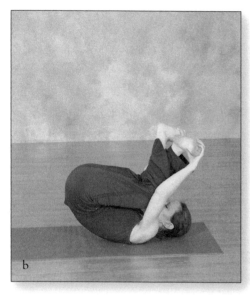

Inhale, rolling back

Practice Off the Mat

Notice the subtle changes happening in your life. Do you sleep better after yoga practice? Are you more aware of your breath and how it relates to your emotions?

The next time you are in a tension-causing situation, consciously relax your shoulders and establish your diaphragmatic breath. Notice the positive effects of actively working stress out of your body.

Wise Words

Learn what every posture has to teach you.

Listen to the sound of your breath, feel it in every cell, and imagine that the breath is stretching you.

Every emotion leaves an imprint on the physical body.

Softening the Edges

Intention

To train the body and mind to surrender to the practice.

Approximate Time

2 to 3 minutes

Lesson

Lie in shavasana. Take a few minutes to relax and settle the body, especially the abdominal area. Then gently focus your attention on your breath.

Allow your breath to be loose and unrestricted. With each exhalation, let the weight of your body surrender to the floor. Allow every muscle to release its grip on the bones. Feel your eyes relax and soften, and allow your facial muscles to release.

During today's practice, keep the definition of yoga, or union, at the top of your mind. This is about being integrated and connected to your breath, body, and mind. From this integration comes liberation, and that's when yoga happens.

The breath leads this connection. By staying linked with the breath, we may direct prana, or life force, into areas that are tight, shallow, or shut down. We can then slowly and mindfully build an asana out of the breath's vibration, letting the breath move us.

When you work with this purpose, the pose then becomes alive, easy, and fluid, not forced, stiff, or breathless. Tight edges gently soften.

Roughness or shortness of breath is a symptom that you are forcing things instead of softening first and letting the breath do its job.

Instead of trying to first get yourself into an asana, first get into the breath and then flow with it into the asana. Let your breath be your partner. Become one with it.

Let's try it. Follow your in-breath and out-breath. Connect with the breath before you begin to move your body.

Asanas for Deepening

During the reclining side stretch, soften the ribs and each side of the back in order to help relax into the postures that follow.

For the twisting triangle, stand with feet three to four feet (about one meter) apart. Line up the toes and heels. Bring one hand toward the floor and reach toward the sky with the opposite arm. Twist, using your hips and arms to deepen. Spread your shoulder blades wide. Soften the pose one breath at a time. Welcome the subtle openings from hamstrings to shoulders and from heels to fingertips.

During the standing yoga mudra, enjoy pouring your body toward the floor. Drain the tension from the shoulders and upper back.

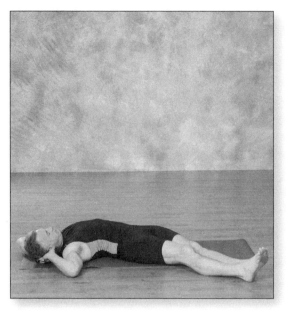

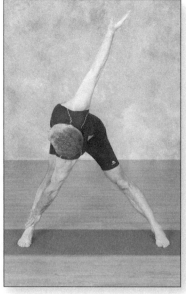

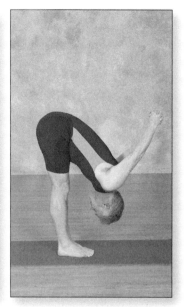

Reclining side stretch   Twisting triangle   Standing yoga mudra

Practice Off the Mat

Every time you say something negative to yourself, it has a tiny but measurable negative effect on your body. Think about what you think as well as what you say.

Wise Words

Keep your postures inventive. Re-create them over and over, if necessary.

Give your muscles permission to soften and lengthen.

Accept where you are in this moment. Acceptance is the ingredient that will make change possible.

Make your lines long. Then lengthen those lines without collapsing or making the pose stiff or dull.

Acknowledge rather than resist your limitations. Tell yourself, "It's okay to be just who I am."

Body Tension

Intention

To discover the roots of tension.

Approximate Length

3 to 4 minutes

Lesson

Today, through breath and body awareness, we'll work with and through body tension.

From the yogic perspective, every tension has a cause. Ask yourself what's causing you to be tense today. Where do you hold this tension?

Tension can originate from anything: relationships, work, anger, fatigue, caffeine, sugar, even something that happened many years ago that still lingers. Muscle tension blocks the natural flow of lymph, hormones, nerve impulses, blood, and pranic energy. Eventually, these blockages affect other parts of the body, creating weaknesses and lowering resistance to disease and infections.

It's the ripple effect.

Tension may also be caused by excess. We can overdo things such as food, exercise, work, even rest. We can spend too much time doing something or in the presence of someone we don't like. The key is to discover our needs for balance in our lives—or at least what balance means to us today.

Our yoga practice teaches us how to use our body tension as a learning tool to guide us into the areas of ourselves that we feel we need to work on.

Let's now lie down in shavasana. Tune into the body on the ground. Feel the parts of the body that touch the ground. Pay close attention to the breath. This can be difficult because if the mind is busy, it's moving much faster than the breath. The breath may feel awkwardly slow compared to the speed of your thoughts. Acknowledge this without judgment. Keep practicing.

In your mind's eye, gently look inside for the tight areas. Explore where you hold tension and what may be causing it. If your shoulders and neck are tight, ask them why. Keep your eyes closed and let your mind open up. A few simple words or visuals may come to you. Take the time to look clearly at what's there.

Asanas for Deepening

Practice approaching poses with tension. For instance, go into trikonasana (triangle) with exaggerated shoulder tension, then consciously remove the tension. Naukasana (boat) releases a central acupressure point located between the navel and the breastbone. Long, deep breathing in this pose helps free body tension. Shoulder openers release tension in the shoulders and upper back. During gomukasana (cow's face), feel the hips settling to the ground. Frustration and anger are often lodged in the hip area.

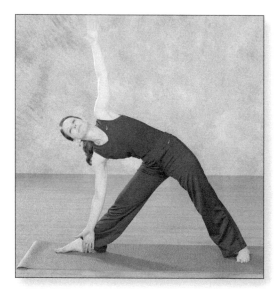

Trikonasana

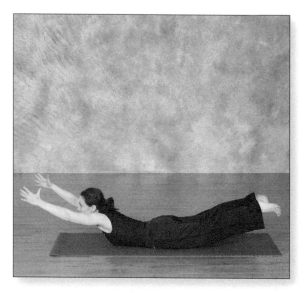

Naukasana

Shoulder Openers

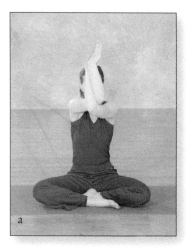

a

Eagle arms

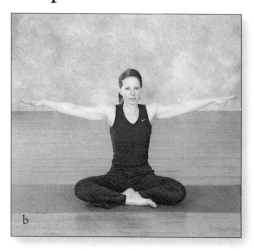

b

Arm swing wide

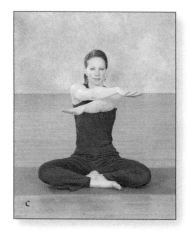

c

Arm swing across

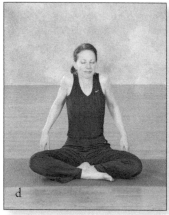

d

Shoulders tense

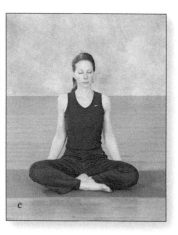

e

Shoulders release

Neck Rolls

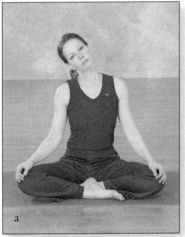
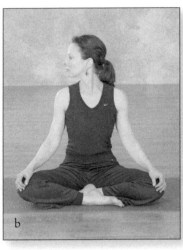
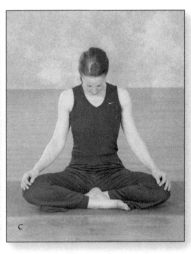

Ear to shoulder   Look over shoulder   Chin to chest

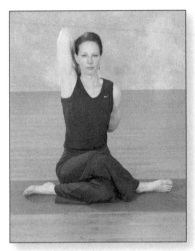

Gomukasana

Practice Off the Mat

Be open and receptive to other benefits of yoga, benefits that may come at any time during your day.

Watch your anger. Uncontrolled emotions can use up a great deal of energy. A few minutes of anger can cost more energy than a day of physical labor.

Wise Words

The pose should feel bright and light; otherwise it becomes heavy and clogged.

Once you choose to let go of tension, you make room for change to happen.

The wise man lets go of all results, whether good or bad, and is focused on the action alone.

Lengthening the Exhalation

Intention

To learn the art of relaxation during stressful life situations.

Approximate Time

3 minutes

Lesson

[Begin class with neck and shoulder rolls.] Lie in shavasana. Take a few minutes to relax and settle the body. Then gently focus your attention on your exhalation, following the exhalation all the way down into the pause at the end of the breath. Calmly focus on watching your breath for a few minutes.

With each exhalation, feel the weight of the body surrender to the floor, allowing every muscle to release its grip on the bones. Then very gradually lengthen your exhalation. If you feel any shortness of breath, back off a bit. The extension of breath should feel natural. Open your mouth if this helps.

Continue until you find a comfortable rhythm that makes you feel relaxed and calm. As you enter a deeper state of relaxation, let go of any control of your breathing and simply watch the spontaneous breathing pattern that's now happening.

Notice how you feel. Does the mind feel clearer? Do the muscles feel relaxed? Note that this ability to willfully relax is only a few exhalations away.

In today's practice, let's use this gift of lengthening the exhale to facilitate healing.

Asanas for Deepening

Notice the cleansing power of the exhalation within each asana. For adho mukha shvanasana (downdog), move into the posture with a long exhale, squeezing the navel toward the spine. For janu shirshana (head to knee), exhale and fold forward. Do this several times. As you inhale, feel the chest opening and lifting away from the pelvis. Discover any tight or stuck spots and breathe into those places, releasing tension with the out-breath. For parivrtta utkatasana (twisting chair pose), begin in chair pose with legs together. Bring the palms together at the heart, twist to one side, and then place one elbow on the outside of the opposite knee. Continue to drop the pelvic bones in order to experience relaxed effort.

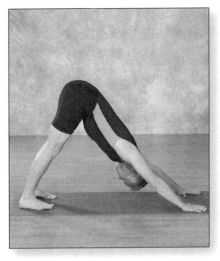

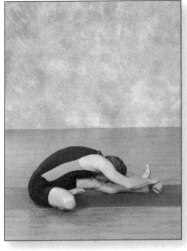

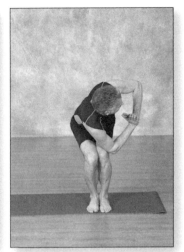

Adho mukha shvanasana   Janu shirshana   Parivrtta utkatasana

Practice Off the Mat

During stressful times, take long, conscious exhalations and feel the tension leaving your body, along with toxins, darkness, and unwanted emotions.

Wise Words

Not knowing how long we are going to stay in a pose forces us keep our attention on the moment, a practice that leads to a sense of peace and happiness.

By being attentive to thoughts and sensations, we come to understand that the mind constantly influences asana.

Scan your body and find out where you feel stuck or open, strong or weak.

Defining Ha and Tha

Intention

To define hatha yoga.

Approximate Time

2 to 3 minutes

Lesson

The balance of body, breath, mind, and spirit is not an easy one. From day to day, minute to minute, we may find ourselves emotionally swinging back and forth. But when we're able to calm the body and mind, we can more readily accept and adapt to life's changes and challenges. This is an essential component to living a more satisfied, joyous, and balanced life.

Fundamentally hatha yoga is about balance. The definition of yoga is union, yoking, or joining together. Ha means sun and tha means moon—opposites—and all the attributes that go with these opposites: hot and cold, dark and light, physical and mental, left and right, male and female. Hatha yoga is the union of opposites in order to reach mental, physical, and spiritual balance.

It is the physical practice of executing particular postures with proper breathing, which then leads to harmony among body, breath, mind, and spirit.

The ancients tell us that the postures were originally developed as a prerequisite to dharana (concentration) and dhyana (meditation). To the ancient yogis, the body was seen as a vehicle to the soul, and meditation was the key to getting there. But in order to sit in meditation for long periods of time, the body must be free of tension and flexible enough to sit without discomfort. The mind should be quiet and able to concentrate.

The body is the vehicle to the soul, so treat it with respect. Feel your boundaries. Sense your limitations. On all levels of consciousness, however, expect and allow yourself to expand, to get better, and to experience a calm heart.

While seated or in shavasana, bring all your awareness to your breathing, establishing the diaphragmatic breath. Feel your abdomen rise and fall with each breath. Observe the natural flow of breath in and out of your body. Let the breath be the link between the mind and the body.

Asanas for Deepening

Remember to balance the ha and tha by combining easy with challenging, relaxing with invigorating, stretching with strengthening.

For the serpent, press the toes toward the forehead. While stretching, note the difference from one side to the other.

During vrikshasana (tree), notice the difference in balance between left and right.

The hatha flow moves from trikonasana (triangle, photo *a*) to parivrtta trikonasana (revolving triangle, photo *b*) to parshvottanasana (angle, photo *c*). Focus on one side at a time. Feel the effects of left versus right or stronger versus weaker. Are you feeling warm on one side? Off balance on the other?

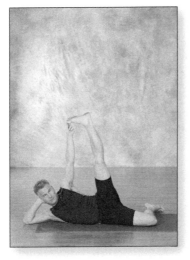

Serpent

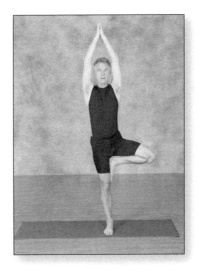

Vrikshasana

Hatha Flow

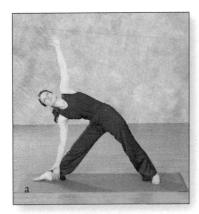

Trikonasana

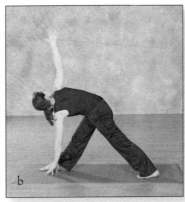

Parivrtta trikonasana

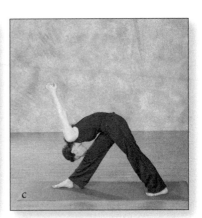

Parshvottanasana

Practice Off the Mat

To find pleasure in yoga as well as in life, we have to focus on what we are doing, one thing at a time. Live the moment.

Wise Words

A posture isn't a posture unless you're breathing through it and thus connecting with it.

You can't measure the quality of your yoga practice on the depth of your forward bend or the flexibility of your hamstrings. It's not about how your postures look; it's how they feel.

While we practice, keep in mind that combining the breath and the movement, while having a calm focus, helps free the mind for a deeper awareness of the moment.

Lengthen your subtle lines of energy by visualizing filling them with light, air, and intention.

When a posture becomes effortless, it becomes meditation.

Chapter 2
Breathing Practices

To keep the body in good health is a duty. Otherwise we shall not be able to keep our mind strong and clear.

—**Buddha**

This chapter will further your practice and teaching of complete breathing. At the core, these are the finest tools for better health, better living, and better awareness.

In all of the lessons, being able to establish the complete diaphragmatic breath is key. If the breath is shallow or uneven, these exercises will be nonproductive and may cause dizziness or lightheadedness.

Focusing the breath is a decision to live in the moment. Let us take a mindful breath as we embark on the training for a yogic life.

Two-to-One Breathing

Intention

To live a more relaxed life even during stressful times; to feel the power of the exhalation during asana.

Approximate Length

3 to 5 minutes

Lesson

Lie in shavasana. Gently leave your past and your future. Keep your attention in the now: the feeling of your body on the ground, the sound of my voice, the awareness of your breath. If your attention is focused, then your mind is also focused.

Let your breathing be free and easy, and establish your diaphragmatic breath. Watch your abdomen rise and fall.

When we feel stress in either the body or the mind, our breathing becomes shallow and we breathe from the chest. This causes our inhalation to be longer than our exhalation, which in turn causes toxins and tensions to build up, making us vulnerable to more anxiety.

The simple process of two-to-one breathing lengthens our exhale so that it's twice as long as our inhale. This quickly calms us down, releases mental tension, and induces a natural state of relaxation.

Let's try this now by gently slowing down the exhalation until we're exhaling to a mental count of four and inhaling to a count of two. Pull in the abdomen slightly to get a longer exhalation. Don't force the breath on either the in-breath or out-breath. We're simply changing the rhythm of breath. [Pause one to three minutes.]

Return to normal diaphragmatic breathing.

We'll use this two-to-one breath in many of our asanas today, so it's important to pay attention to the quality and length of your breathing.

Asanas for Deepening

Practice any standing or seated forward bend such as parshvottanasana (angle) or baddha konasana (butterfly) using two-to-one breathing. Observe how the torso moves and loosens with each exhale. Also notice your level of patience and mental clarity. For the woodchopper, use a long exhale as you visualize chopping the wood between your legs.

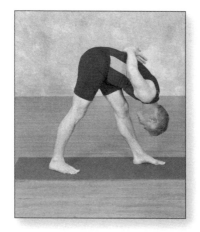

Parshvottanasana

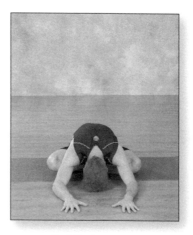

Baddha konasana

Woodchopper

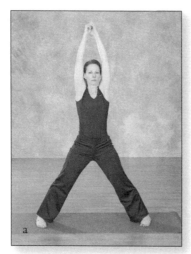

a

Arms above head

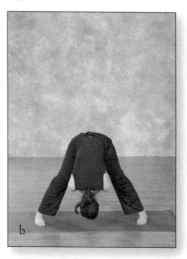

b

Arms between legs

Practice Off the Mat

The technique of exhaling as long or longer than you inhale helps to release stress, allowing you to act instead of react.

Counting the length of breath at any time during the day is a useful method of practicing dharana, or concentration.

Wise Words

Each breath is like an ocean wave swelling and contracting.

Notice that when you get distracted, it shows up in your breathing.

Continually challenge yourself to stay mindful.

Three-Part Exhalation

Intention

To enhance exhalation and stimulate a deepening of inhalation, which are beneficial for releasing built-up tension.

Approximate Length

3 to 4 minutes

Lesson

Today we'll consciously alter our breathing pattern so that we can directly experience how this changes our thinking patterns. We'll lengthen the exhalation by dividing the exhalation into three equal parts, pausing briefly between each exhalation.

This produces a longer exhalation than you might normally take. The three-part exhale is useful if you have trouble falling asleep or getting rid of anxiety or for those times when you have a buildup of tension, which is common during menstruation and menopause.

Begin by taking a normal breath in, and then divide your exhalation into three equal parts so that you empty the breath from the top of the torso to the bottom, from throat center to pubic bone.

Breathe like this: Inhale completely, then exhale from the throat to the heart. Pause, then exhale from the heart to the navel. Pause, then exhale from the navel to the pubic bone. Pause, then inhale completely again. Let each part of the exhalation be of equal length. The pauses between the sections of exhalation should feel like a calm moment of hesitation rather than a feeling of holding the breath.

Take a couple of normal breaths in and out then repeat the three-part exhalation. You may imagine each exhalation as a soft leaf falling slowly down to earth, gently touching the tree branches at each pause until it reaches the ground. Or visualize walking down a tall staircase, exhaling as you step down, pausing at each step before descending further. Or you may just want to visualize the breath moving from collarbones to heart center, heart center to navel center, navel center to pubic bone.

Try about 10 breath cycles, then relax.

Asanas for Deepening

For each asana, use the three-part exhalation to help you with the pose.

During the seated twists (simple twist, photo *a*, or marichyasana, photo *b*), use the three-part exhale to move into the pose. As you do this, feel how the exhale strengthens the depth of the pose.

For prasarita padottanasana (spread-leg forward bend), use a three-part exhale to take the pose downward. Note how a relaxed breath helps to relax and brighten the pose itself. Inhale and fill your posture with breath. Exhale and melt the crown toward the ground.

As you come out of setu bandha sarvangasana (bridge), release the backside with a three-part exhale, feeling each section of vertebrae touch the earth.

Seated Twists

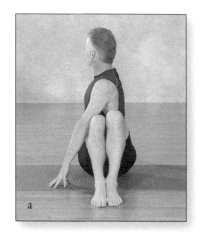
a

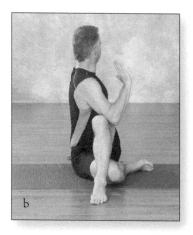
b

Simple twist

Marichyasana

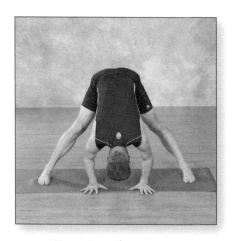

Prasarita padottanasana

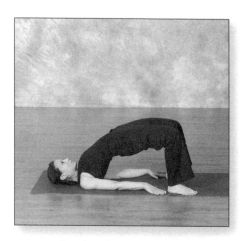

Setu bandha sarvangasana

Practice Off the Mat

Consider your time on the mat as a means to sweep through your energy field, erasing both mental and physical debris. As in weeding a garden, you are cleansing and creating more space for growth. Feel the lightness as you allow the mindfulness of yoga practice to lift the weight of your worries from your consciousness.

Wise Words

A focused mind directs prana.

When you can direct your prana, you are in charge of your own lifeforce.

If we are filled with toxins, tensions, and closed-down body parts, how will we find room to store prana?

Stretch the breath as long as you can.

Ujjayi Breath

Intention

To bring a deeper awareness of the postures by internalizing attention.

Approximate Length

3 to 4 minutes

Lesson

Today we'll learn ujjayi breath. Unlike regular diaphragmatic breathing in which the throat is relaxed and the breath is silent, ujjayi uses an audible vibration with purposeful tension.

This type of breathing during asana, or during some pranayamas, soothes the nerves and calms the mind. The sound naturally draws attention to the breath and internalizes awareness. It also helps develop awareness of subtle body and psychic sensitivity. Using ujjayi during asana practice is an excellent preparation for meditation.

Ujjayi requires breathing against the resistance of a constricted glottis, which is the aperture in the throat that opens and closes when you hold your breath. It's just behind the Adam's apple. The closing of the glottis allows pressure to build up before you cough and closes when you hold liquid in your mouth as you gargle.

Ujjayi has a distinctive sound. It sounds a little like ocean waves. [Demonstrate the breath, walking around to each student so that they can hear.] The breath is deeper than normal. The easiest way to deepen the breath is simply to expand the abdomen fully during inhalation and to contract it completely during exhalation.

To learn this, whisper "ha" with the mouth open on the exhale and whisper "ah" on the inhale. Then gradually close the mouth. You should begin to feel the glottis or the air on the back of your throat.

You may notice a short pause in the sound of ujjayi after inhalation and exhalation, but don't allow a pause in the breathing itself. Each inhale flows into the next exhale.

Be attentive to the soothing effects on the mind and the nervous system. We'll work with ujjayi during most of our asana practice.

Asanas for Deepening

Ujjayi leads to a deeper awareness of the posture by internalizing the attention.

For padmasana (lotus pose), breathe ujjayi and feel the breath move up and down the spine. Mentally repeat the mantra of the sound of the breath. Inhale, feel the breath move down the spine, and mentally repeat *so*. As you exhale, mentally repeat the sound *hum* as the breath moves up the spine.

For the lunge series, work with long, deep ujjayi breaths through a selection of lunge variations, including deep hip openers such as lunge with heel to hip (photo *a*) and lunge with elbows on the ground (photo *b*).

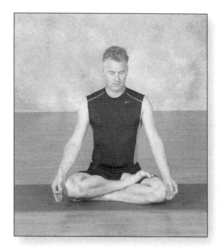

Padmasana

Lunge Series

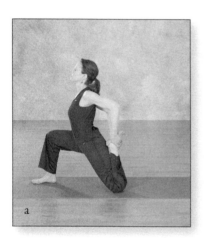

a

Heel to hip

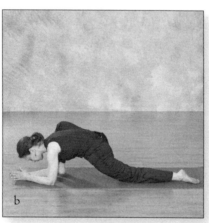

b

Elbows on ground

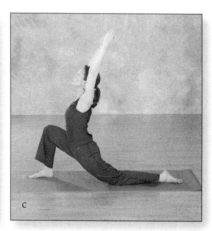

c

Back knee down, arms up

Practice Off the Mat

Allow life, like a yoga pose, to unfold naturally. Resist the temptation to dominate the situation or the body.

As with each breath, experience the newness of now.

Wise Words

Ujjayi promotes the internalization of the senses.

As the breath becomes more refined, so does the posture.

Be patient with yourself if you forget ujjayi after only a few breaths. Continued practice will allow you to keep track of both the posture and the breath.

Ujjayi is a combination of two Sanskrit words: *ud*, which means up, and *jayi*, which means victory.

Nadi Shodhana

Intention

To teach alternate-nostril breathing and its benefits.

Approximate Length

8 to 10 minutes

Lesson

[This lesson can be practiced at the beginning, middle, or end of class.] Our pranayama practices are meant to control prana, the vital energy within us. There are over 72,000 nadis, or subtle energy channels within the body through which prana moves. If the nadis are blocked, prana doesn't move freely through the body, which inhibits consciousness and makes it difficult to find meaning in daily life. This can result in the manifestations of suffering: distraction, dullness, anger, fear, anxiety. But as the nadis are purified—cleansed—prana can travel freely and consciousness is awakened.

Nadi shodhana is a breathing exercise that helps purify the nadis, focusing most directly on the two main nadis, the pingala and the ida. Pingala ends at the right nostril; ida ends at the left.

Pingala, the right nostril, embodies the sun and has a heating effect on the body. It's linked to left-brain function and is associated with active external energy, intellectual pursuits, and rational reasoning. It also has a warming effect on the body. When this nostril is open, the pathways to logical thinking are open too. This could be a good time to take a math test or make a business presentation. It gives us the warming power to digest food as well.

Ida, the left nostril, represents the moon and has a cooling effect on the body. It's linked to internal energy and to the right side of the brain. It's connected to imagination, intuitive thinking, and subjective decisions. When this nostril is open, it's the right time for thinking creatively, writing poetry, listening to music, or painting.

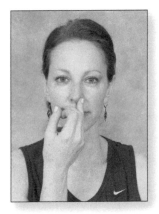

Pingala breathing
(right nostril)

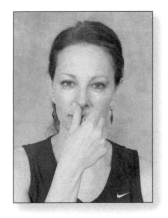

Ida breathing (left nostril)

In nadi shodhana, we alternate our breath between the right and left nostrils, seeking to balance the energies of the sun and the moon. When the nadis are cleared and energies are balanced, prana flows more smoothly.

Let's try one round together. Sit in a comfortable seated position, with your head, neck, and trunk in alignment. Breathe into each nostril separately in order to see which one is flowing more smoothly. Chances are you will have an active nostril and a passive nostril. Begin your practice on your active side. Establish a natural diaphragmatic breath.

Bring the right hand to the nose. Fold the index finger and middle finger so that the right thumb can be used to close the right nostril and the right ring finger can be used to close the left nostril. Inhale through both nostrils.

Close the passive nostril and exhale completely through the active nostril.

Inhale through the active nostril slowly and completely. At the end of the inhalation, close the active nostril, then slowly and completely exhale and inhale through the passive nostril.

Repeat this cycle of exhaling and inhaling two more times.

At the end of the final inhalation through the passive nostril, exhale through both nostrils and take three very deep breaths. This completes one round.

To sum up one round of nadi shodhana, do the following:

1. Exhale active
2. Inhale active
3. Exhale passive
4. Inhale passive
5. Exhale active
6. Inhale active
7. Exhale passive
8. Inhale passive
9. Exhale active
10. Inhale active
11. Exhale passive
12. Inhale passive

Asanas for Deepening

Each nostril relates to different physiological aspects of our being. After practicing a series of deep backbends such as setu bandha sarvangasana (bridge), bhujangasana (cobra), or ustrasana (camel), which are typically very stimulating, check to see if the right nostril is active. Do the same for passive hold poses such as seated forward bends like malasana (garland) or balasana (child's pose). After the hold, check to see if the left nostril is active.

Finally, check the nostrils at the end of sushumna class. Aim to have smooth and open air flow through both nostrils so that sushmna, the central main nadi that runs along the spine and ends at the crown chakra, is activated.

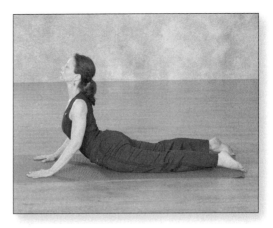

Setu bandha sarvangasana

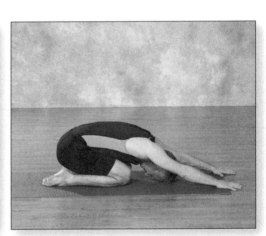

Bhujangasana

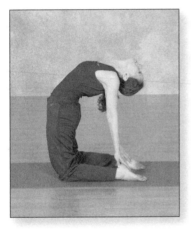

Ustrasana

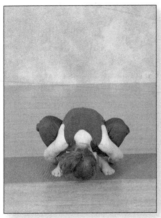

Malasana

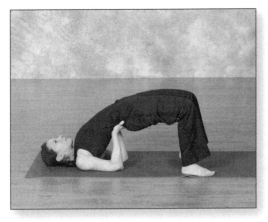

Balasana

Practice Off the Mat

Practice nadi shodhana anytime you need to quiet and calm the mind. Alternate nostril breathing is recommended twice a day. Try it once and you'll feel its effects immediately.

Think of nadi shodhana as a light in the midst of a storm. I knew a student who, during a heated business meeting, excused herself to go the ladies room to practice nadi shodhana. She came back feeling refreshed, clear, and courageous enough to tackle the rest of the meeting.

Practice nadi shodhana to alleviate insomnia, beginning the practice on the left (moon) nostril.

Wise Words

Once you affirm that you are exactly where you want to be and that you are doing exactly what you want to be doing at this moment, you'll be amazed at how much energy is suddenly within you.

Listen to the sound of your breath. Feel it in every cell. Imagine that the breath is stretching you.

The more awakened the pranic field, the more energetic we feel.

Opening the Left Channel

Intention

To open the left nostril and thereby activate the right brain.

Approximate Length

3 to 5 minutes with breathing practice

Lesson

Do you ever come to class feeling agitated or unclear?

When we begin our practice in a relaxed manner, it encourages the right hemisphere of the brain—the side that handles music, color, complex memory, images, and holistic thinking—to function more fully. The right side of the brain then integrates more readily with the left hemisphere, the side of the brain that handles rational thinking, external energies, and heat-inducing activities such as digestion.

There are two main channels of energy—the ida (left) and pingala (right)—that weave lifeforce through the chakras in the spinal column. They end in each nostril. When the breath is carried predominately through the left, prana flows through the channel that keeps the body calm and the mind quiet but alert—the ideal setting in which to practice asana and meditation.

Today we'll begin our practice by opening the left nostril, the nostril that's responsible for activating the right brain. Lie down on the right side, resting your right ear against the inner side of your upper arm. Stay here until the left nostril clears.

Each breath is like an ocean wave, swelling and receding in perfect rhythm. Our yoga practice affords us the time to concentrate on this vital flow of nourishing air into and out of our bodies. Visualize a slow-rolling ocean wave as you breathe completely and effortlessly.

Practice Off the Mat

This practice will quickly alleviate anxiety arising in the body or mind. With the right thumb closing off the right nostril, breathe out of the left nostril, taking three to six complete breaths. Then stop and breathe out of both nostrils for three complete breaths. Repeat the practice until the left nostril is active. You will feel an agreeable shift in consciousness.

Wise Words

The first step in releasing stress is to recognize when you're *feeling* stress. Then, learn the practices that lessen your stress and use them.

Every time you see a red light or long line, instead of allowing yourself to feel burned by impatience, use your time to practice breathing in and breathing out. Smile.

Chapter 3

Asana

Your body is precious. It is your vehicle for awakening. Treat it with care.

—**Buddha**

Asana, the third limb along the royal path, is a powerful, intelligent, and efficient physical practice. Simply by choosing to engage our internal intelligence, we can more clearly advance our healing by penetrating deep layers of consciousness through the body.

Open your mind to creativity within your postures. For instance, if you find that there's a new feeling in trikonasana when you turn your arm this way or that, share it with your students and fellow teachers. The deeper you delve into the process of self-discovery, the more inspiring, natural, and alive the practice and teaching will become.

Guide the way.

Feet

Intention

To practice feeling the body's foundation and to run the earth's energy through it.

Approximate Length

3 to 4 minutes

Lesson

[Begin the class in tadasana, mountain pose.] Do you know how important your feet are? The average person takes 10,000 steps a day. The feet are our foundation. If our foundation is weak, problems may arise in the rest of the body. Many aches and pains in the lower legs, the back, and even the shoulders can be traced to issues in the feet.

In all of the standing poses, the feet—the part of the body that touches the ground—forms the foundation of the pose. If the foundation of a house is out of alignment, the walls will be crooked and might crack. In asana practice, if the feet are misaligned or if the body weight is off center, it will be difficult to strike a tall, spacious, and centered pose.

The weight of your body should be evenly distributed between the outer and inner foot and between the heel and ball of the foot.

As you stand here, become aware of the four corners of the foot: the base of the big toe, the base of the little toe, the inner heel, and the outer heel. If the inner foot feels heavy, the arch may be collapsing. If the outer foot is heavy, the arch of the foot may be high, the base of the big toe may be lifting and the outer ankle could feel strain. Take a moment to feel your foundation and make adjustments if you need to.

To make a strong, well-balanced foundation, the arch should feel lifted and light, while the inner heel and base of your big toe stay grounded.

Let's use this foundation consciousness in our postures today.

Asanas for Deepening

Begin in tadasana (mountain pose). Spread your toes and snuggle the soles of your feet to the earth. Let the weight of your body sink downward into the ground. Feel the openings rise up to the crown of the head. As the weight of the body goes down, the inner feeling rises up.

In all standing poses, from trikonasana (triangle) to virabhadrasana (warrior), notice the position of the feet. Feel the lightning bolt of energy rising up from the ground and coming in through the soles.

For vrikshasana (tree), much of the work is done before the raised foot is lifted off the ground. Begin by establishing the balanced action of your right arch, ankle, and toes in tadasana (mountain). Imagine a root extending from each of the four corners of the right foot down into the earth. From that root system, lift up from the arch of the foot and visualize the pranic pathway through the leg to the pelvic floor and from the pelvic floor through the spine to the crown of the head. Finally lift the left foot and place it on the right leg.

Sit on the toes. The toes are curled down toward the floor, providing a refreshing and much needed stretch for the soles of the feet.

For baddha konasana (butterfly), bend forward and aim the forehead toward the toes. According to ancient teachings, the feet are symbols of humility and peace. Bringing the head, the seat of the ego, and the feet together cultivates more humble and introspective characteristics within our personalities.

The tennis-ball or golf-ball massage is remarkably effective for tired feet and sensitive soles (souls!). While standing, roll a tennis ball or a golf ball under the soles of your feet to stimulate circulation of the foundation.

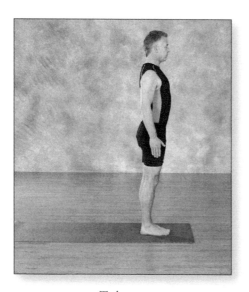

Tadasana

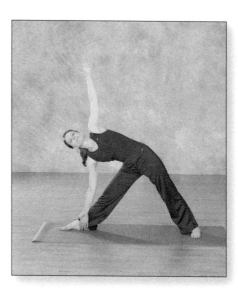

Trikonasana

Virabhadrasana

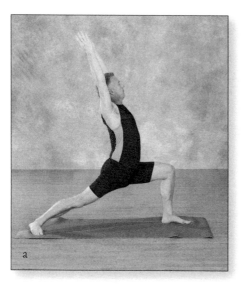

Warrior I

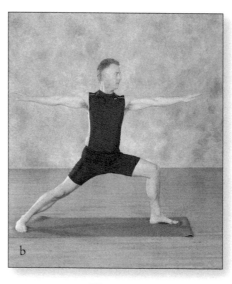

Warrior II

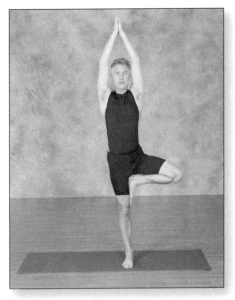

Vrikshasana

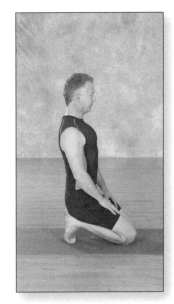

Sitting on toes

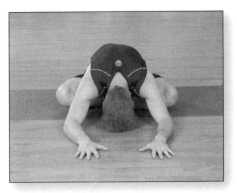

Baddha konasana

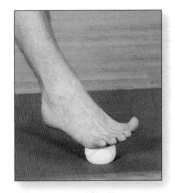

Tennis- or golf-ball massage

Practice Off the Mat

Walk barefoot whenever you can, spreading your toes frequently throughout the day. If you can't walk barefoot, pamper your feet by wearing comfortable shoes.

Reflexology meridians connect all the organs and glands in the body and culminate in the feet and hands. By applying pressure through massage you can send lifeforce and healing to the corresponding area.

Wise Words

Practice breathing easily in all standing poses, securing your foundation.

Feel earth energy coming in through the feet, moving up the legs, and settling in the pelvic floor. From there, make the pose more open and spacious by spreading the pelvic-floor energy through the rest of the body.

Keep the feet active through your practice. Extend the balls of the feet forward and spread the toes. Use as much of your feet as you can.

If any of your toes overlap, separate them with your fingers.

Forward Bends

Intention

To develop a quiet and patient mind through the settling effects of forward bends.

Approximate Length

2 minutes

Lesson

Forward bends are quieting and settling, and they bring us inward, which makes them effective counterposes to the more vigorous backbends. And because they're an excellent antidote to anxiety, they require and develop an infinite amount of patience, perseverance, and humility.

Forward bends stretch and lengthen the spine, the muscles of the lower back, the pelvis, and the legs. The upper back, kidneys, and adrenal glands are stretched and stimulated as well. Forward bends are excellent for relieving mild back pain.

The influences of the mind are observed throughout our entire practice, but forward bends, especially sustained forward bends, are important for understanding that the integration of yoga takes more mental than physical effort.

When you hold a forward bend, you become aware of the melodramas inside your head. Test your patience. See if you can wait out those little mind performances until they drop away completely.

[Be sure to balance the forward-bend sequences with backbends and twists.]

Asanas for Deepening

Paschimottanasana (posterior stretch) is the ideal asana for examining the ebb and flow of the mind. Rather than taking the pose all at once and folding completely to your limit, practice patience by first emphasizing the length of the front torso then slowly bend forward and gradually deepen the pose with breath. Watch it unfold from the inside out.

Try variations on uttanasana (standing forward bend): palms to the ground (photo *a*), hands to the ankles (photo *b*), opposite hand to opposite elbow (photo *c*). Continue letting go again and again using the power of the breath.

For balasana (child's pose), bring the hands to the feet with your palms up. Hum your exhalation on every other breath.

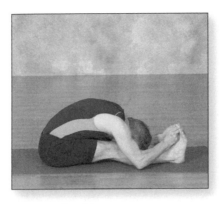

Paschimottanasana

Uttanasana

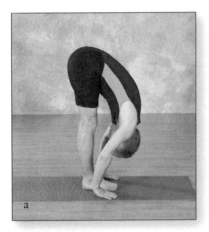

Palms to the ground

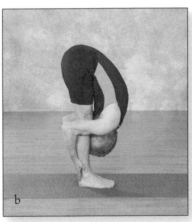

Hands to the ankles

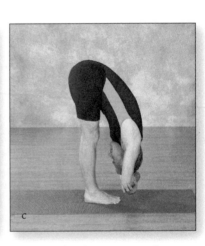

Opposite hand to opposite elbow

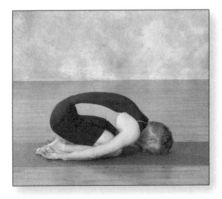

Balasana

Practice Off the Mat

Forward bends help us remember the middle way: not too much, not too little. Whether you are deciding what to eat for lunch or how to behave toward an unfavorable colleague, notice the equilibrium your yogic lifestyle brings you as you practice this philosophy of balance.

Honor your boundaries in life, but expect them to expand. Have fun and have faith!

Wise Words

Paschimottanasana has been called "the stretch of the West." This describes the ancient ritual of yogis facing the sunrise as they practiced. Yogis literally stretched the west side of the body as they bent toward the sun.

Recognizing what is true for you can be difficult if you want to be at a place you aren't ready for.

Explore any negative mental patterns you're bringing to the asana, such as an urge to push or a tendency to let the mind wander.

Backbends

Intention

To understand the physiological aspects of backbends.

Approximate Length

2 to 3 minutes

Lesson

Yoga is defined as restraining the fluctuations of the mind. Our practice is intended to reduce these fluctuations in the frontal lobe of the brain, the part that's most involved in conscious thought.

Our time on the mat is spent moving from the familiar to the somewhat obscure, from the front part of the brain to the back of the brain, and from the front of the body—the known—to the back of the body—the unknown.

Today we are going to bring this awareness to our backbends. As we know, forward bends are quieting and settling, and backbends are just the opposite—they're stimulating and exciting. Backbending asanas bolster a sense of openness, confidence, and bravery. They open the chest, abdominal organs, and pelvic region, basically the whole front side of the body.

Yoga is about oneness and integration of body, mind, and spirit. So when areas in the body—front, back, or side—are closed down, it makes us feel more separate, and it limits energy flow. This can cause mild depression, fear, and weakness.

The physical aspects of backbending work counter to these impressions because they improve circulation along the spine, helping to relieve depression and other symptoms of feeling closed off. Ultimately they leave us feeling confident, refreshed, and alive.

[Be sure to balance backbends with forward bends, twists, and neutralizing poses such as balasana (child's pose).]

Asanas for Deepening

Before beginning the backend, lengthen the pose first, and then explore the depth. Depth without length creates constriction. Even and steady breathing, with a focus on completing the exhalation, inhibits overstimulation of the sympathetic nervous system. This makes for a calmer pose. Because backbends can be difficult to deepen and explore on your own, these postures allow for exceptional and expansive adjustments by a teacher or partner.

Practice a series of asanas in order to work up to chakrasana (wheel), such as standing backbend, both supported (photo *a*) and unsupported (photo *b*) bhujangasana (cobra), urdhva mukha shvanasana (updog), ustrasana (camel), dhanurasana (bow), inverted table, and setu bandha sarvangasana (bridge).

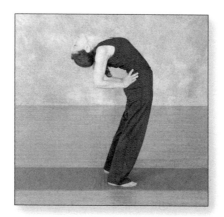

Standing backbend

Bhujangasana

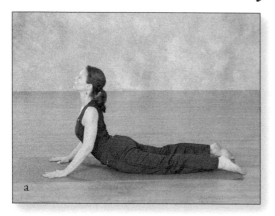

a

Supported

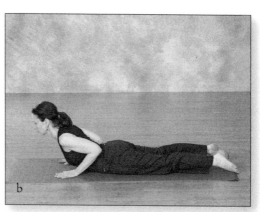

b

Unsupported

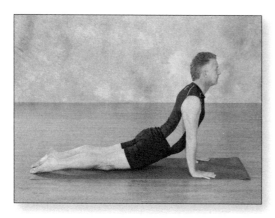

Urdhva mukha shvanasana

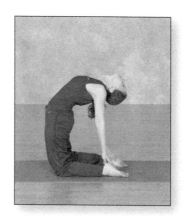

Ustrasana

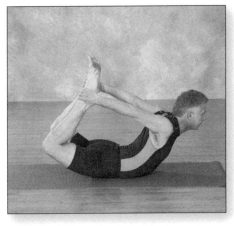

Dhanurasana

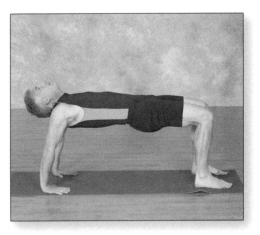

Inverted table

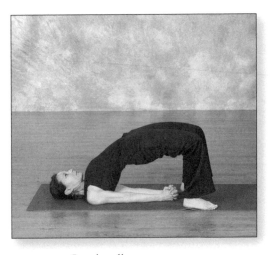

Setu bandha sarvangasana

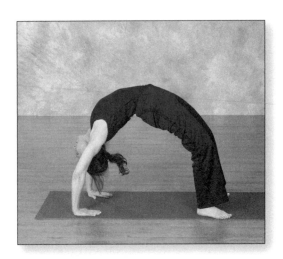

Chakrasana

Practice Off the Mat

Simple backbends, such as unsupported cobra and bridge, are recommended for anyone with breathing difficulties such as asthma. They can be exhilarating, creating openings in the chest, ribs, and collarbone areas, consequently allowing inhalation to flow more freely. They are also beneficial when you feel sluggish and need a quick pick-me-up asana.

Wise Words

The power of backbends is subtle, yet immediate. They work directly on the nervous system, which is why they help ease mild depression.

Backbends are a bit mysterious and provocative because they engage a part of the body you can't see.

Let the posture be the tool that allows you to hold more energy, more light. Make room for your spirit to be free.

Twists

Intention

To learn to twist properly so that the body and mind receive a squeeze-and-release cleansing effect.

Approximate Length

3 to 4 minutes

Lesson

Today our focus will be on twists. The twist is the great equalizer: if you are tired, they pick you up; if you are anxious, they help calm you down.

The virtue of the twist is that it wrings out the body and assists in releasing tension. When we release the twist—the wringing-out action—and the muscles relax, the areas that were involved in the twist become flooded with nutrients and fresh blood.

Twists tone and cleanse your organs, release and strengthen the muscles of your spine and neck, and allow you to open and strengthen your shoulder joints.

As the torso rotates, the kidneys and abdominal organs are activated and exercised. This improves digestion and removes sluggishness. Since every nerve begins in the spinal cord, every part of the body rejuvenates, heals, and becomes more vital. We become more comfortable in our bodies and more inspired with life force.

Let's discuss the physical principles of the twist by taking a simple seated twist in easy pose, pelvis in a neutral position.

Put your awareness at the crown of your head. Open the crown so that the chest, neck, and head are lifted. Then elongate and align the spine by pressing your sit bones into the floor. Bring your left hand to your right knee and your right hand behind you. Inhale and lift. As you exhale, gently rotate to the right from the base of the spine up through the low back, waist, shoulder blades, and finally neck. With every breath, continue to lengthen the spine, which creates space in the vertebrae and brings about a deeper and safer experience.

These principles will be included in all of the twists we'll be practicing today.

[Remember to balance your twist practice with forward and backward bends.]

Asanas for Deepening

Begin with the reclining twist. Allow your rib cage to release and your feet and knees to settle to the earth. Move into seated twists: simple twist (photo *a*) and marichyasana (half spinal twist, photo *b*). Next perform garudasana (eagle). Most twists focus on the torso, but garudasana benefits both the legs and the arms. For parivrtta trikonasana (revolved triangle), twist from the base of the spine and continue up to the crown of the head. Finish with a runner's lunge twist with namaste.

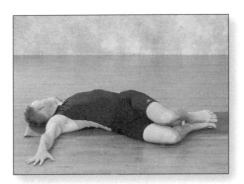

Reclining twist

Seated Twists

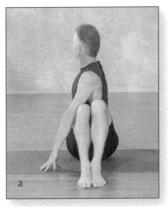

a

Simple twist

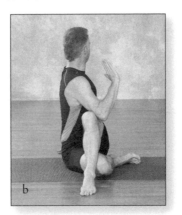

b

Marichyasana

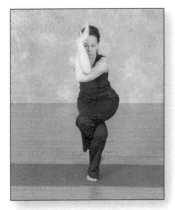

Garudasana

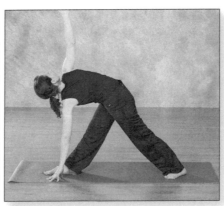

Parivrtta trikonasana

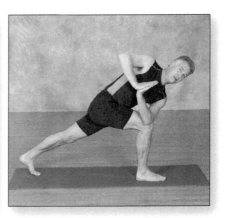

Runner's lunge twist with namaste

Practice Off the Mat

If you spend a lot of time in a chair, take several twist breaks during the day. Bring your knees to one side of the seat and your hands to the arm you are twisting toward or to the back of the chair. Extend upward on your inhale. On your exhale, gently twist to the side your knees are facing.

Wise Words

Twists keep avidya—or spiritual tunnel vision—out of our lives. By staying present with everything around us and in back of us, we keep our inner vision clear and unobstructed by illusion.

Twists allow us to stay present during life's changes.

Before you begin the actual twisting movement, lengthen your torso as much as you can by pressing downward and reaching upward. Feel the spine come to life.

Headstand

Intention

To enjoy the benefits of the king of asanas.

Approximate Length

2 to 3 minutes

Lesson

Shirshasana, or headstand, is known as the king of asanas because it has legendary benefits, including increased vitality, improved concentration, and enhanced glandular function.

Accomplishing headstand, however, can be a significantly challenging achievement. Some of us have trouble with it because we either don't have enough strength and flexibility in our shoulders and hamstrings or we have weak lower backs and abdominal muscles. Fortunately a number of preparatory asanas address these problems.

A third hurdle may be the most overlooked. Headstand requires overcoming the anxiety and fear of turning upside down and possibly falling. For those of you in this category, please use the wall for support.

Contraindications for practicing headstand include high blood pressure, heart problems, cervical-spine injuries, detached retina, glaucoma, osteoporosis, neck injuries, excess weight, pregnancy, and menstruation.

Let's begin the headstand with some postures that lay the groundwork for the king of asanas.

Asanas for Deepening

Some schools of yoga counter headstand with tadasana (mountain pose), while others follow with balasana (child's pose) to alleviate any dizziness. Trust your inner teacher, and stay connected with what feels best for you.

Practice these preparatory postures before demonstrating headstand:

- The reclining hamstring stretch opens the hips and hamstrings.
- The lunge series consists of a lunge with the back knee on the ground (photo *a*) and a lunge with the elbows on the ground toward the inside of the front foot (photo *b*). (A simple runner's stretch can be included as well.)
- Unsupported bhujangasana (cobra) develops the low-back muscles.
- The fire series (leg-lift series) strengthens the navel center. Include bicycling (photo *a*), spread-leg stretch (photo *b*), and double-leg lifts (photo *c*).

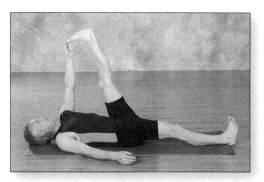

Reclining hamstring stretch

Lunge Series

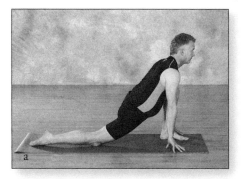

Lunge with back knee on ground

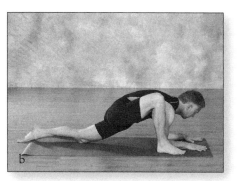

Lunge with elbows on ground

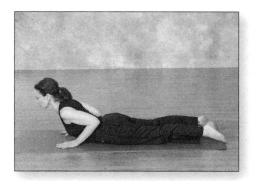

Bhujangasana

Fire Series

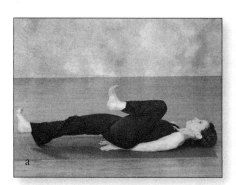

Bicycling

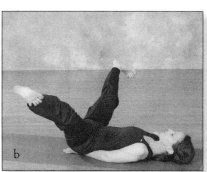

Spread-leg stretch

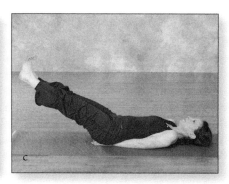

Double-leg lifts

- For shoulder stretches, include eagle arms (photo *a*), cow's-face arms (photo *b*), and arm swings (photos *c* and *d*).
- Dolphin is the consummate pose for preparing for headstand. Dolphin develops strength and flexibility in the shoulders as it strengthens the abdominal and back muscles.
- Setu bandha sarvangasana (bridge) opens the upper chest and stretches the spine. Hands are interlaced beneath the spine. The tops of the shoulders are rolled under.
- Halasana (plow), sarvangasana (shoulder stand), and matsyasana (fish) are the last three preparatory asanas.

Shoulder Stretches

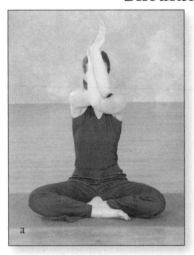

Eagle arms

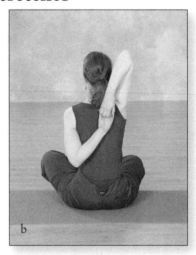

Cow's-face arms

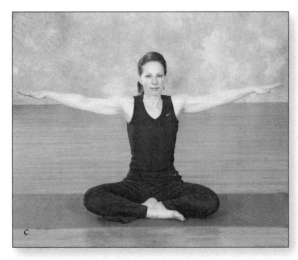

Arm swings, arms open

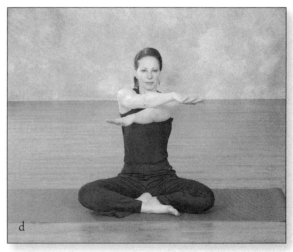

Arm swings, arms crossed

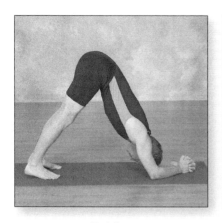
Dolphin

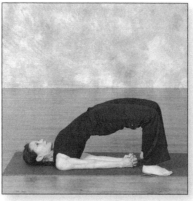
Setu bandha sarvangasana

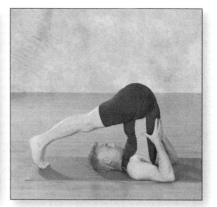
Halasana

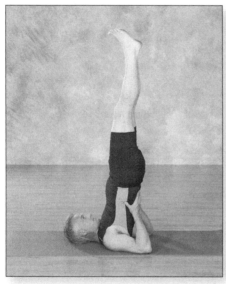
Sarvangasana

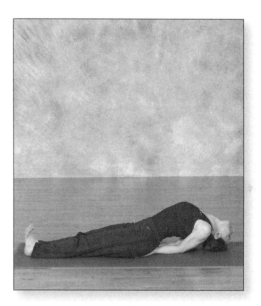
Matsyasana

Shirshasana (headstand) requires a slow start and demands an impressive amount of core and shoulder strength. First lift the knees to the chest and collect your balance (photo *a*). Then straighten your legs, lifting the soles of the feet up to the sky (photo *b*). Keep the weight of the pose on your forearms rather than on the crown of the head. Breathe! As you build strength, try the tripod variation (photos *c* and *d*) as you learn headstand.

Shirshasana

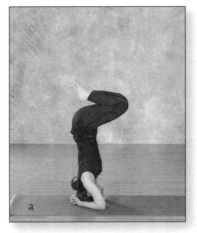

Halfway up

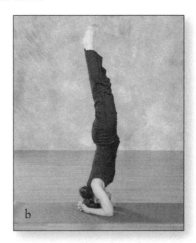

Full headstand

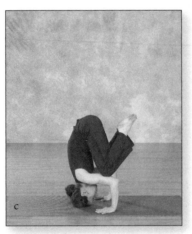

Tripod, knees on upper arms

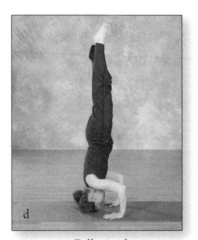

Full tripod

Practice Off the Mat

Keep thinking positively. Allow yourself to be guided from within.

Notice the confidence and inner strength that's revealed when headstand is practiced.

Headstand stimulates the crown chakra, our connection to divine spirit.

Wise Words

If balance changes as you raise your legs slowly up into headstand, stop moving until you gain equilibrium.

Moment-to-moment awareness is the secret to balance.

Deepen your headstand by adding ujjayi breath. Ujjayi is effortless in inversions because the throat is already compressed.

If you can remain in headstand for just three minutes, the blood will drain to the heart and tissue fluids will flow more efficiently into the veins and lymph channels of the lower extremities.

Asana and Acceptance

Intention

To study Patanjali's definition of asana; to accept where we are in asana as in life.

Approximate Length

2 minutes

Lesson

In Patanjali's *Yoga Sutras*, asana is defined as a pose that is both steady and comfortable. In this sense, the interpretation means to be fully present, to be exclusively alive to the now experience.

Learning to be present and to participate in anything that is both steady and comfortable means freeing yourself of any thought or sensation that allows space for the suffering experience such as self-judgment. When you live this way, you are practicing yoga. You are living thoroughly.

Many times in our practice—and in our lives—we respond from a place of judgment. "I can't do this posture" or "Everyone else is more flexible than I am" or "This posture doesn't make any sense!"

Our practice is to abandon criticism for the next hour. If you do criticize something or someone, just notice the judgment, then check to see if it is placed on your emotions, your body, or your breath. Then let it go.

Today, if you find yourself forcing in asana, or in any other part of your life, ask yourself, *is this the true spirit of the practice of yoga*? When things are steady and comfortable, there is no forcing.

Asanas for Deepening

Teach postures that you and your class may find challenging, such as ardha chandrasana variation (half moon with foot hold), tittibhasana (firefly), or yoganidrasana (yoga sleep pose). Break down the postures into practice postures. For ardha chandrasana with ankle hold, use a strap around the back foot. With tittibhasana, practice lifting one leg at a time. And in yoganidransana, try putting one leg at a time behind the arm or shoulder.

The practice is not to **perfect** these poses but to feel the potential ease and comfort that is possible anywhere in any asana when you practice acceptance.

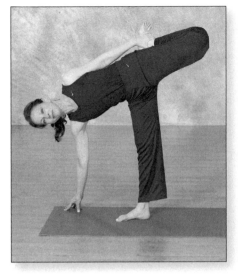
Ardha chandrasana variation

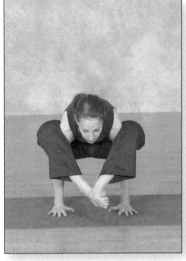
Tittibhasana

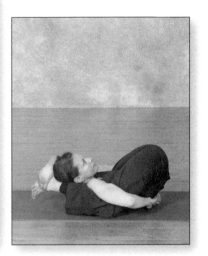
Yoganidrasana

Practice Off the Mat

Take a look at your life. Notice areas that you'd like to be different or eliminated entirely, places that do not feel steady and comfortable. Can you make adjustments in your mind-set as you do in your asana? Allow these areas in your life to flow through you so that you can accept rather than agonize.

Feel yourself becoming sensitized and responsive. Consciously put passion into your life, and sense the heightened perception.

When things are forced, it feels like we're attempting to put a square peg in a round hole.

Wise Words

Don't worry about what anyone thinks. The problem with craving acceptance is that it puts the power base outside of yourself.

Accept where you are in this moment without striving, without comparing, and without judging.

Go where it feels the most desirable, where your energy flows best. You have the ability to sense this. Trust it.

Everyone has a different idea of what *steady* and *comfortable* mean. What do they mean to you today?

Asana is not what it looks like from the outside; it's what it feels like on the inside.

If there's a place in your body or an aspect of your emotions that need extra attention, invite that energy to surround those areas of your life without judgment.

Asana and Peace

Intention

To learn that yoga practice can have a positive impact on peace.

Approximate Length

2 minutes

Lesson

Those of us who practice yoga benefit from nonviolence and a peaceful spirit. Our asana practice brings about a peaceful frame of mind because it asks us to become more sensitive, more conscious, and more aware of ourselves as bodies, minds, and spirits. This awareness makes us clearer and calmer, more awakened to truth and thus better able to handle life's endless challenges.

As we become more awakened, we move away from forcing and controlling events, and we move toward letting the universe take care of many of our daily dilemmas. In turn these changes influence the consciousness and actions of everyone we meet. The sensitivity we develop on our yoga mats affects everyone around us.

You soon begin to see and notice that slowly, yogi by yogi, we can shift the direction of the world.

Asanas for Deepening

The parrot (half squat, half lunge), symbolizes neutrality, one who takes action without analysis, repeating what others say without attachment.

In the clam (easy pose with forward bend), experience the wonder of being breathed. Who is in control of this breathing? It happens 24 hours a day, every day, for your whole life, without conscious effort. Now breathe awareness into your muscles. Don't let the breath get blocked along the way.

Finish with the peaceful-warrior flow series, moving from virabhadrasana II (photo *a*) to virabhadrasana I (photo *b*) to virabhadrasana III (photo *c*). Practice using the intuitive feeling of courage. Be bold. Feel the fortitude, the firmness, the determination it takes to practice the postures. Dare to confront the difficulties of life with a peaceful intent to face internal conflicts head on.

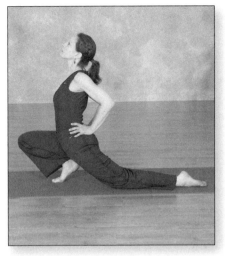

Parrot

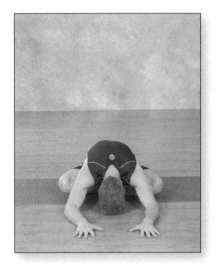

Clam

Peaceful Warrior Flow Series

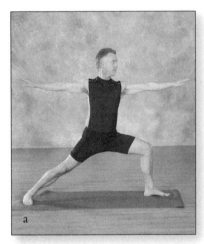

a

Virabhadrasana II

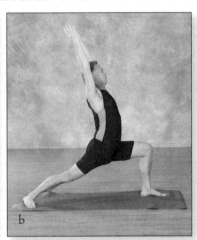

b

Virabhadrasana I

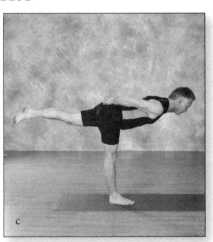

c

Virabhadrasana III

Practice Off the Mat

The moment we start to force a situation (this can be especially true during times of impatience and desperation), we begin to lose awareness of our nervous system and the truth of the circumstance itself. This will inevitably create struggle and discomfort. Breathe thoroughly and look for peace in every situation.

Wise Words

Forcing the body past the point of resistance is an act of self-aggression and is the opposite of practicing peace.

Spread peace wherever you go.

The surest way to be happier is to do all you can to improve the lives of others.

Chapter 4
Salutations in Motion

However many holy words you read, however many you speak,
what good will they do you if you do not act on them?

—Buddha

In yoga practice, the salutation may be interpreted as vinyasa, or asana-linked breath. In the context of this chapter, salutation refers to a movement of gratitude toward our universe: our sun, our moon, our earth, ourselves. By acknowledging the connection of mind and body, salutation becomes a way we demonstrate our appreciation for the forces of life that are given to us, the forces that ultimately animate and complete our existence.

The salutation is not limited by planets or by nature. Create your own salutation in the form of honoring your students, children, parents, home, even the food you eat. Indeed through space and movement, these practices celebrate the wondrous attributes of all living things.

Surya Namaskara (Sun Salutation)

Intention

To create awareness of the physical and spiritual benefits of sun salutation.

Approximate Time

3 to 4 minutes

Lesson

Surya namaskara, sun salutation, is the graceful sequence of postures executed as a continuous, flowing motion. The postures are linked with the breath. Each asana counterbalances the one before it, stretching the body and elongating the spine forward and backward. These movements alternately expand and contract the chest to regulate the breathing.

On the physical level, sun salutation is frequently used to warm the body for the more challenging postures that follow. But it is foremost an invocation to honor the life-giving energies of the sun.

To many practitioners, sun salutation is performed as a prayer to commemorate our inner light. It shows devotion to the external sun, the creative life force of the universe that yogis believe radiates both inside and outside the body.

Sun salutation begins with a focus on gratitude, with the inner eye turned inward to the spiritual heart. Filling your heart with awareness and appreciation for what the sun provides—internally, externally, and symbolically—transforms these postures from mere exercises into an act of devotion toward all aspects of nature.

To practice the sun salutation with an attitude of gratitude, visualize the sun rising and setting day after day for millions of years. Visualize it lighting, beautifying, and warming the environment, while supplying the necessary elements to grow food. Connect with this visualization by feeling the heat around your body, and notice the energy that radiates a few feet around your body. Before we begin our first round of salutations, draw that sun energy into your heart and let it illuminate within you.

Asanas for Deepening

Sun loops. When we lift the arms in the sun, we open ourselves to the universe.

1. Bring hands to the heart in anjali mudra (prayer position, photo *a*).
2. Inhale and reach the arms up and over the head (photo *b*).
3. Exhale and burst your hands apart (photo *c*), palms up until shoulder height, then palms down, moving hands toward thighs (photo *d*), then back to anjali mudra.
4. Perform with a swift, heat-generating movement. After doing three to five sun loops, pause long enough to feel the "loops" of heat around your body and then feel them gradually rest in the heart center.

Sun Loops

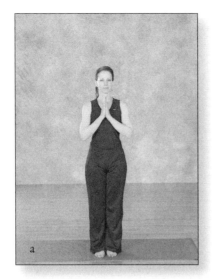

Hands to heart in anjali mudra

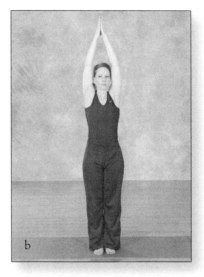

Arms reach over head

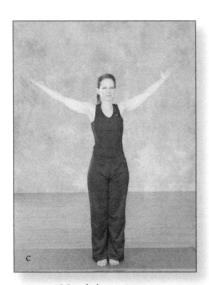

Hands burst apart

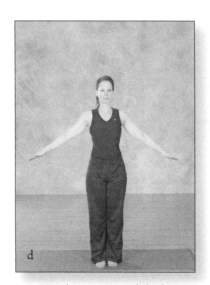

Hands move toward thighs

Surya namaskara. The sun salutation stretches and strengthens every major muscle group. Move through the sequence in a continuous, flowing motion leading with the breath.

1. Tadasana (mountain) with hands in anjali mudra (prayer position).
2. Tadasana (mountain) with arms overhead (photos *a* and *b*).
3. Uttanasana (forward bend, photo *c*).
4. Lunge (photo *d*).
5. Plank (photo *e*).

6. Bhujangasana (cobra, photo *f*).

7. Adho mukha shvanasana (downward dog, photo *g*).

8. Lunge (photo *h*).

Surya Namaskara

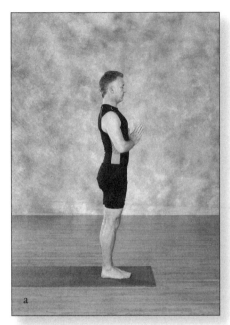

a

Tadasana, hands in anjali mudra

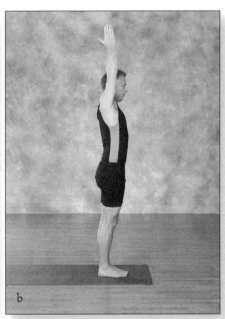

b

Tadasana, arms overhead

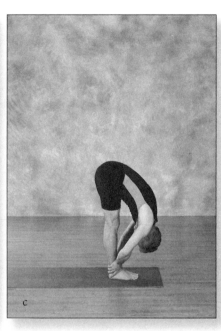

c

Uttanasana

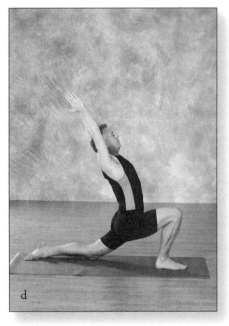

d

Lunge

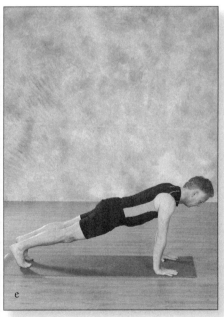

e

Plank

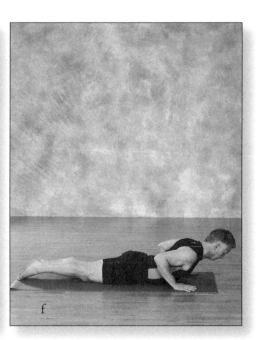

f

Bhujangasana

9. Uttanasana (forward bend, photo *i*).

10. Tadasana (mountain) with arms overhead (photo *j*).

11. Tadasana (mountain) with hands in anjali mudra (prayer position, photo *k*).

Surya Namaskara *(continued)*

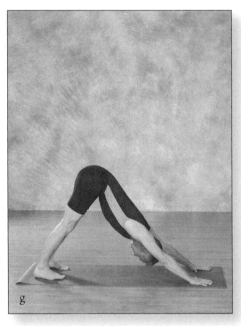

Adho mukha shvanasana

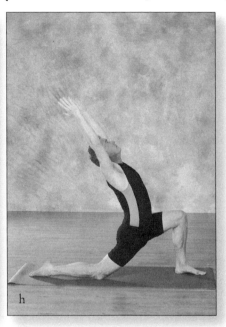

Lunge

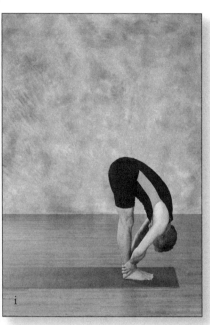

Uttanasana

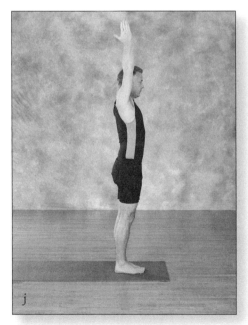

Tadasana, arms overhead

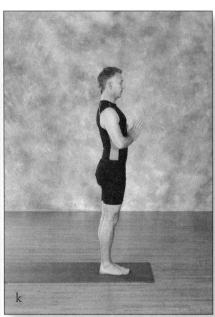

Tadasana, hands in anjali mudra

Practice Off the Mat

At sunrise, thank the sun for its life-giving powers and be grateful for this new day.
Watch the sun set, and thank the sun for another blessed day on earth.

When the sun is hidden on a cloudy day, remember that the sun is a constant. It is always there to take care of the universe.

Wise Words

The outer sun is a representation of our inner sun; it corresponds to the subtle or spiritual heart.

The ancient yogis describe the heart as the only place in the subtle body that knows the truth; the practice of sun salutation unleashes the truth of the deeper self within the heart.

The Sanskrit word *surya* means sun. *Namaskara* is the Hindi word for *namaste*, from the root *nam*, to bow.

Chandra Namaskara
(Moon Salutation)

Intention

To connect with the cooling, female energy of the moon.

Approximate Time

3 minutes

Lesson

Chandra namaskara, moon salutation, is a powerful equalizer to sun salutation. While sun salutation heats up the body, utilizes our male-orientated and external energies, and emphasizes pingala, the right nostril, moon salutation acknowledges the inner self in order to discover our lunar, cooling, female energies associated with ida, the left nostril.

Moving through the two salutations in one practice, even alternating between the two, helps fulfill the ideology of hatha yoga: the sun (ha) and moon (tha) coming together as one in an effort to balance the opposing parts of our conscious and unconscious spectrum.

The phases of the moon represent the growth, maturation, and death cycle that all things must experience. Each phase of the lunar cycle has its own personality, and each is expressed within the human body. The waxing phase, from the new moon to the full moon, represents the growth stage. The waning phase, from the full moon to the new moon, correlates to the flowering, fruiting, and dying within our consciousness.

Moon salutations cultivate a calming, rejuvenating quality and are said to be most beneficial when practiced at night when the moon is visible. We'll begin with several rounds of sun salutation in order to heat the body and activate our external forces. We will then follow with moon salutation to balance our energies.

Asanas for Deepening

To establish harmony after experiencing too much solar energy or during menstruation, try the restorative postures supta baddha konasana (reclined bound angle) and supported upavistha konasana (supported open angle). Use blankets or bolsters beneath the torso to bring in cooling energies and open the lower belly and pelvic floor.

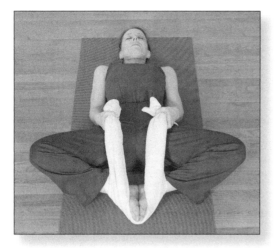

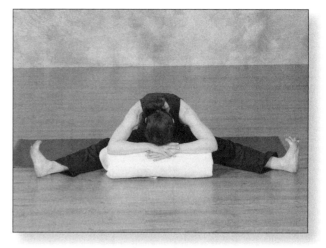

Supta baddha konasana   Supported upavistha konasana

Chandra namaskara. The moon salutation cools and calms the nervous system. Repeat the salutation on both sides. Visualize the moon in a clear night sky, shining brightly overhead.

1. Tadasana (mountain, photo *a*), palms pressed together in anjali mudra (prayer position).
2. Side moon (photo *b*). Interlace fingers and then point your index fingers up in temple position. Lean to one side and then to the other.
3. Victory squat (photo *c*).
4. Five-pointed star (photo *d*).
5. Trikonasana (triangle, photo *e*).
6. Parshvottanasana (angle, photo *f*). Lower both hands toward either side of the foot on the ground.
7. Lunge (photo *g*). Release back leg to the ground.
8. Extended-leg squat (photo *h*). Walk hands to the center. Take back leg into squat and lengthen front leg forward.
9. Squat (photo *i*).
10. Extended-leg squat (photo *j*). Extend opposite leg.
11. Lunge to opposite side (photo *k*). Release back leg to the ground.
12. Parshvottanasana (angle) to opposite side (photo *l*).
13. Trikonasana (triangle) to opposite side (photo *m*).
14. Five-pointed star (photo *n*).
15. Victory squat (photo *o*).
16 Side moon (photo *p*).
17. Tadasana (mountain, photo *q*).

Chandra Namaskara

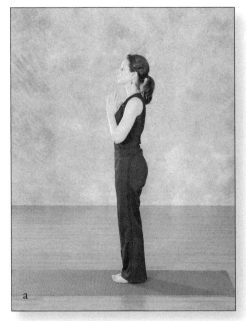

Tadasana, palms together in anjali mudra

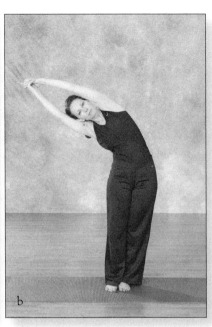

Side moon

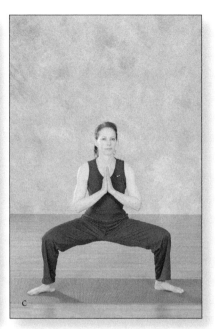

Victory squat

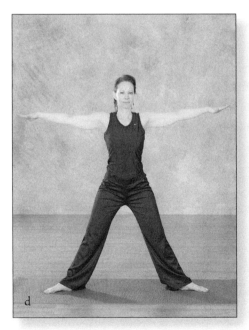

Five-pointed star

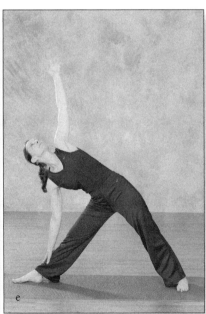

Trikonasana

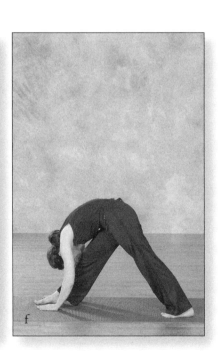

Parshvottanasana

(continued)

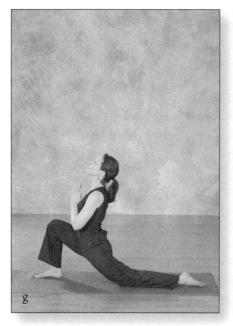

Lunge

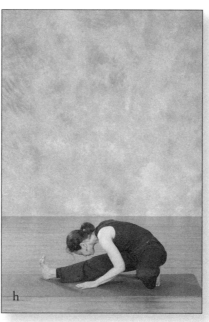

Extended-leg squat

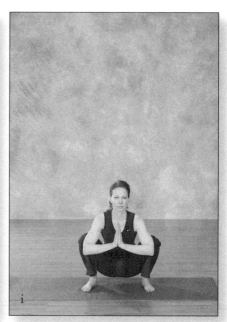

Squat

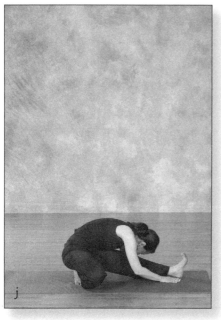

Extended-leg squat

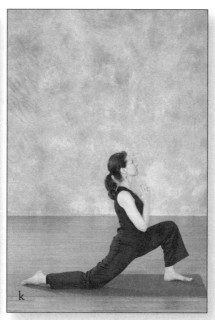

Lunge

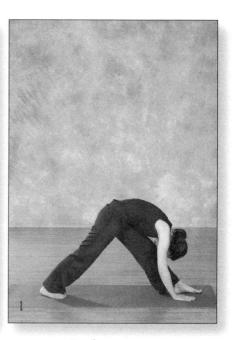

Parshvottanasana

Chandra Namaskara *(continued)*

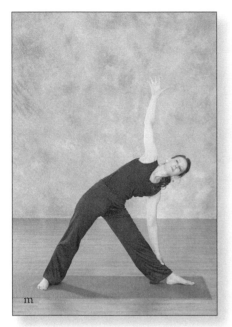

Trikonasana

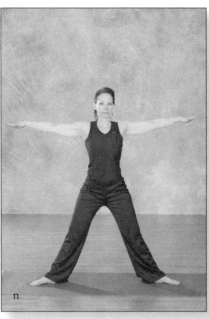

Five-pointed star

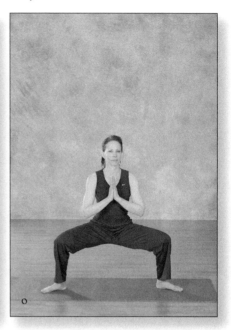

Victory squat

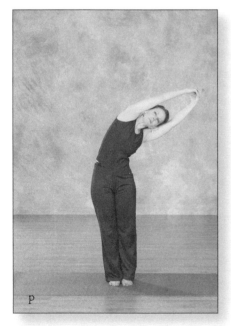

Side moon

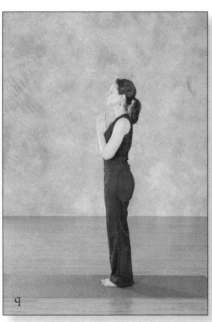

Tadasana (mountain)

Pranayama practice: chandra shodhana. To open the internal lunar energies, close the right nostril with the right thumb and breathe from the left nostril. Begin with one round of six complete breaths. Chandra shodhana is often practiced to defuse stress, anxiety, and mood swings associated with hypertension. (See nadi shodhana on page 28 for an overview of alternate-nostril breathing.)

Chant to the moon. *Aum som somaye namah aum.* Translation: Atman (universal spirit), your moon fills me with passion. I call out to you with love, my Atman.

Practice Off the Mat

In yoga philosophy, full-moon days are called "days of opportunity." If there is something you want to bring into your life, the best time to do it are the during the days between the new moon and the full moon. As the moon grows toward fullness, it is said that the things you desire will grow and come to you. The new moon is a time to take advantage of the growing essence of the tides and begin a new project, career, or relationship.

Wise Words

Just as the tides of the ocean are affected by the phases of the moon, so are the waters—the tides—within our bodies.

The full moon represents the fully awakened mind. The ancient yogis believed that the lunar phase an individual is born under will set a particular tone for their soul's evolution during this lifetime.

Star Salutation

Intention

To learn the king of salutations.

Approximate Time

3 minutes

Lesson

A star is a celestial body that is visible from the earth at night. Stars that are grouped together form galaxies, which make up the universe. The nearest star to the earth is the sun, the main source of energy on earth. Star salutation, which honors our entire galaxy, is sometimes referred to as the "king of salutations."

As we practice star salutation, notice how many of the movements expand the body into the shape of a pentagram. From the physical perspective, we are stretching in all directions, using our arms, legs, and head as the tips of the star. Spiritually, the pentagram has long been associated with mystery and magic, yet it is the simplest form of a star shape. It can be drawn with a single line, so it's sometimes called "the endless knot." For yoga students, this symbolizes the endless energy patterns within us.

Star salutation gives us a tremendous side stretch and helps strengthen the muscles along the torso. Also, unlike the basic sun salutation, star salutation delivers a twist so that we may explore the entire solar system circulating within us. Feel your individual power and remember that every miniscule drop you create in the universal ocean has a ripple effect on everyone around you.

Let's stretch our internal and external universe by learning the star salutation, the "king of salutations".

Asanas for Deepening

Star salutation. Be a star and shine prana to every point in your body. Think of the head, arms, and legs as points of the star. Hold the postures for a minimum of three complete breaths, longer for more experienced students. Repeat the sequence on the opposite side.

1. Tadasana (mountain, photo *a*). Take three centering breaths, remembering your purpose in the universe today.
2. Tadasana (mountain, photo *b*). Lift the arms up toward the biggest star of all, the sun.
3. Uttanasana (forward bend, photo *c*). Reach toward the earth.
4. Five-pointed star (photo *d*). Lengthen, open, and energize the whole body.

5. Victory squat (photo *e*). Turn out the toes, hands in namaste. Lift the ribs off the pelvis and imagine someone pushing down on your thighs, taking your posture deeper. Lift up on your toes, if you like. Bend the knees and bow to the earth. Feel the connection between the cosmos and the earth.

6. Trikonasana (triangle, photo *f*). Visualize triangle as a star tipped to the side.

7. Parivrtta trikonasana (revolved triangle, photo *g*). Move into revolved triangle from triangle without coming to stand.

8. Ardha chandrasana (half moon, photo *h*). The standing foot merges with the floor as you move your feet away from each other.

9. Virabhadrasana III (warrior III, photo *i*). Shine and breathe into your five star-points: crown of head, arms, and legs.

10. Five-pointed star (photo *j*).

11. Uttanasana (forward bend, photo *k*).

12. Tadasana, with arms lifted upward (photo *l*).

13. Tadasana (mountain, photo *m*). Take three centering breaths before beginning on the opposite side.

Star Salutation

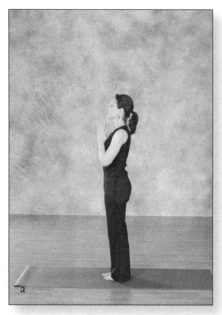

Tadasana

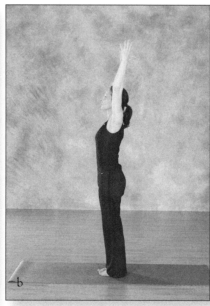

Tadasana, arms lifted toward sun

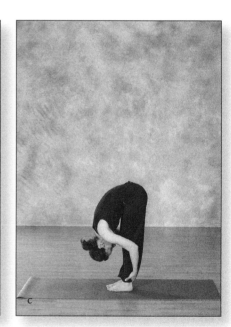

Uttanasana

Star Salutation *(continued)*

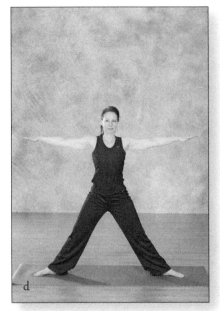

Five-pointed star

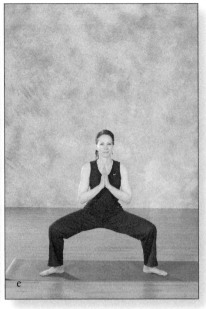

Victory squat

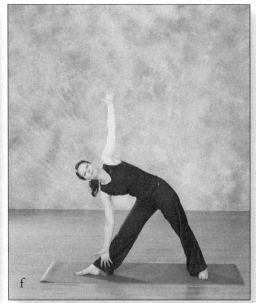

Trikonasana

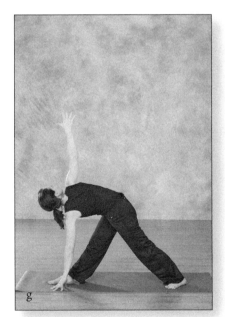

Parivrtta trikonasana

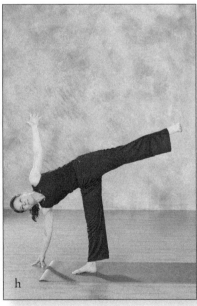

Ardha chandrasana

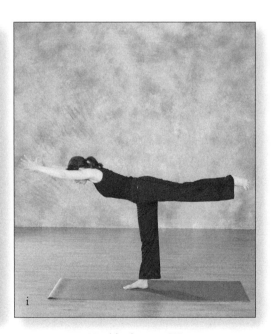

Virabhadrasana III

(continued)

Star Salutation *(continued)*

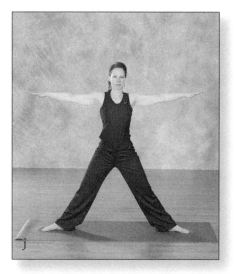

Five-pointed star

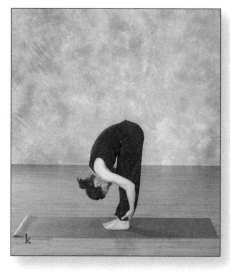

Uttanasana

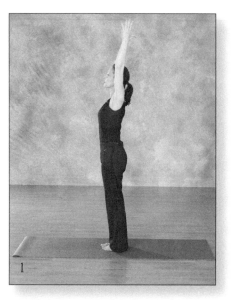

Tadasana, arms lifted toward sun

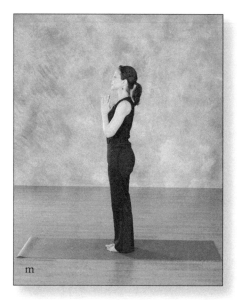

Tadasana

Practice Off the Mat

Off the mat, imagine the head, arms, and legs as the five points of the star, the heart as the center of the star. Feel your life force radiate through you. The more you practice this visualization, the more others will sense your shining energy.

When stars accumulate together, they become a galaxy. Who in your life is part of your galaxy?

Wise Words

As you expand the body, every cell expands and becomes porous.

Connect from the core of your being to the core of the universe.

Visualize everyone in the class forming a small but influential universe.

Earth Salutation

Intention

To experience the grounding effects of the earth salutation through an outdoor practice.

Approximate Length

2 minutes

Lesson

There is much we can learn while coping with the challenges, sensations, and sensitivities of the human body. When we feel that our consciousness is not grounded in our physical form, we become scattered or spacey. When this happens, we can call on Mother Earth to ground us, to use the potent, grounding energy of nature, such as the mountains, trees, and grass. Human beings are tied to the earth, but as yogis, we are constantly unfolding, reaching up to the sky in an effort to both lengthen our spine and feel our connection between heaven and earth. The process of yoga practice begins with feeling our foundation; when we are connected to Mother Earth, we can open ourselves to all spiritual possibilities.

We're going to do that today by taking our practice out-of-doors. The awareness begins at our feet, as it carries the earth's energy up the legs, into the pelvis, and up the spine. If wind, sounds, insects, and birds distract you, know that it's Mother Nature's way of telling you to focus on your practice and bring your awareness back to the earth.

Asanas for Deepening

Earth salutation. While earth salutation can be experienced indoors, the intention is to feel the earth beneath the feet. This practice may be taught on grass or on sand, without the use of mats.

1. Balasana (child's pose, photo *a*). Extend through the arms and touch the earth.
2. Adho mukha shvanasana (downward dog, photo *b*). Inhale and exhale as you rise up on the toes from the initial position.
3. Candlestick (photo *c*).
4. Tadasana (mountain, photo *d*).
5. Vrikshasana (tree, photo *e*).
6. Standing splits (photo *f*).
7. Prasarita padottanasana (wide-leg forward bend), with palms to the earth (photo *g*).
8. Tadasana (mountain, photo *h*).
9. Balasana (child's pose), with hands behind by the hips (photo *i*).

Earth Salutation

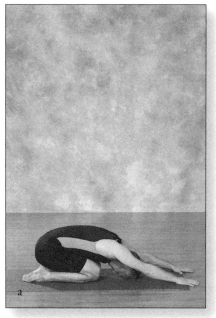

Balasana

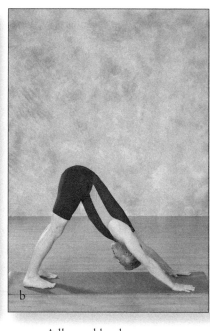

Adho mukha shvanasana

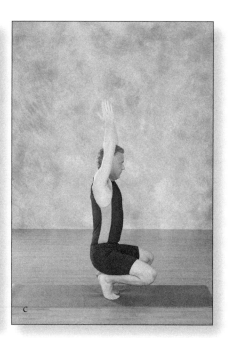

Candlestick

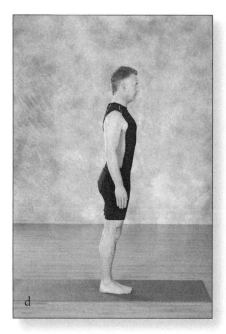

Tadasana

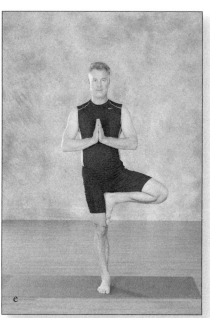

Vrikshasana

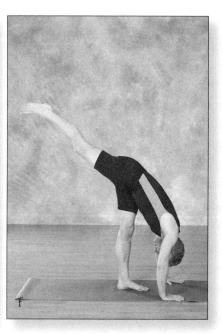

Standing splits

Earth Salutation (*continued*)

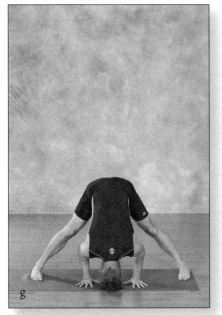

Prasarita padottanasana

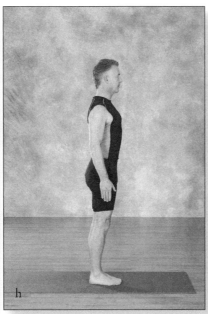

Tadasana

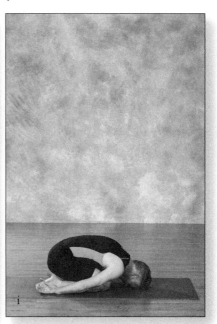

Balasana

Practice Off the Mat

Celebrate Earth Day on April 22 with a nature walk.

Enjoy a walking meditation through the woods, feeling each step synchronize with your breath.

Go to the beach and build a castle, bury your toes, or practice your tree on the sand. Build a sand castle close to the water and watch the surf take it away.

Wise Words

Being wholly present in your body can help you understand how your time as a physical being contributes to your purpose in life.

Practice the earth salutation when you're feeling scattered and unable to concentrate. Visualize the grounding effects of Mother Earth.

In spring and summer, sense the vitality of the earth beneath you. In winter, when the ground is frozen, remind yourself that the earth is in a spiritual slumber until the birth of spring.

Self Salutation

Intention

To honor our own inner light.

Approximate Length

3 to 4 minutes

Lesson

At the core of honoring ourselves and our inner light is self-love. First the heart must be full of compassion for ourselves. Only then will we be able to radiate that beauty out to others.

The path of honoring ourselves begins with self-acceptance. We may fear being judged by our choices, by our character, by how our bodies look. When we accept our feelings, we can experience changes in consciousness. We find fulfillment from within simply by accepting what is present in this moment, without trying to change a thing.

Today we'll practice the self salutation. As we practice, stay present in your body and become aware of the skin, bones, muscles, and all their sensations. Take a deep breath and feel your feet on the floor. Notice the way your ribcage moves as you breathe. Notice how you feel emotionally as well as physically. Remember that outer joy is an extension of the love we have for ourselves. Forget about the things you wish you were and were not, and let's honor ourselves for who we are right now.

Let's begin with a moment of gratitude. Think of all the ways your body and spirit have helped you along your journey, and thank yourself accordingly.

Asanas for Deepening

Self salutation. Feel each asana in your soul and the vibrations of healing in your body. Take the time to allow yourself to fully inhabit your amazing self.

1. Tadasana (mountain), with arms folded (photo *a*).
2. Virabhadrasana I (warrior 1, photo *b*).
3. Virabhadrasana II (warrior II, photo *c*).
4. Parshvakonasana (triangle II, photo *d*).
5. Kapotasana (resting pigeon, photo *e*).
6. Adho mukha shvanasana (downward dog, photo *f*).
7. Yoga mudra, with hands interlaced behind the back, weight on the crown (photo *g*).
8. Balasana (child's pose): Pause in humble adoration of the self (photo *h*).

Self Salutation

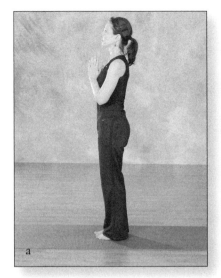

Tadasana

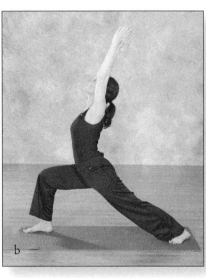

Virabhadrasana I

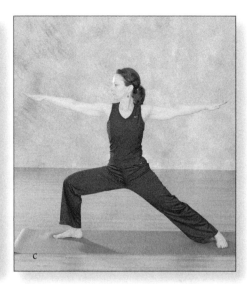

Virabhadrasana II

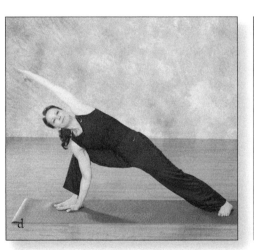

Parshvakonasana

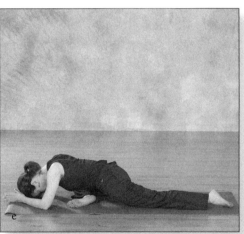

Kapotasana

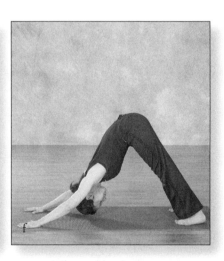

Adho mukha shvanasana

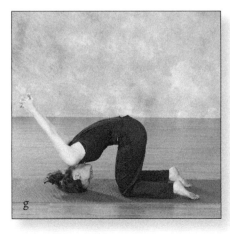

Yoga mudra

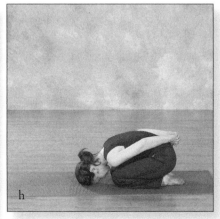

Balasana

Practice Off the Mat

Listen to yourself, including your inner thoughts, when you are in the company of others. Do you criticize your body or spirit more often than you thought? If you catch yourself criticizing your body or actions in any way, send yourself loving, compassionate messages about how special a being you really are.

Learn to enjoy being by yourself. If you rarely get a chance to be alone, set aside a time once a week to be with yourself, your own best friend.

Participate in activities that you enjoy—dancing, walking, making pottery, flying a kite, or cooking. Feel the joy in your body when you do something that feels spiritually invigorating.

Wise Words

Never underestimate the importance of self-acceptance. It can end emotional pain and lead to a lifetime of spiritual enlightenment.

The body is a miracle, and you're inside of it. You are the miracle!

Practice letting go of the activities, people, and ideas that are toxic, heavy, and dark. They will consume your life force.

Love and cherish your body. As long as this vehicle is healthy, let go of doubts and self-criticisms about how it looks.

To be the most compassionate, loving beings we can be, we must be compassionate to ourselves.

Chapter 5
Prana

Thousands of candles can be lighted from a single candle, and the life of the candle will not be shortened. Happiness never decreases by being shared.

—Buddha

A fundamental comprehension of prana can make or break a student's yoga class experience. Prana is defined as anything that animates life both in the body and in the universe. This is referred to as life force.

The complexities of the hatha yoga journey are realized when we understand that the life force that illuminates me also illuminates you, as well as the tree outside, the squirrel in the tree, and the forest floor around the tree.

We get a clearer sense of not only how nature relates to our individual life force but also how we are each a pranically connected wave in the ocean of life.

Holding On to Prana

Intention

To understand the discipline of maintaining pranic balance.

Approximate Length

2 to 3 minutes

Lesson

To understand the holistic practice of yoga, it's important to recognize prana, the energy that we're made of. Prana is a Sanskrit word that can be defined as life force. It signifies the energy that flows through the nadis, the body's subtle energy channels.

The breath is the most significant way we bring life force into our bodies. We also receive prana from food, from sleep, and from emotions such as love and happiness.

But if our emotions are disturbed or if our sleeping and habits are inadequate, our prana can be scattered and our life force lost or wasted. To be strong and healthy, we have to learn how to keep our prana inside the body and how to direct it. We can also learn to restrict the loss of prana during disturbing circumstances.

We often have to step away from negative or draining situations in order to stay healthy. This discipline is vital for holding on to prana. It allows us to retain enough life force to stay focused and balanced. In asana practice, we train ourselves to watch for distractions and interruptions and to notice when we wander off.

In today's practice, notice when the mind wanders and how long it takes to come back to the moment. This is how we begin to feel our life force. We start to see that practice is changing us. Physically, we discover places, such as the shoulders, neck, or hips, where prana is blocked. Through mindfulness, we focus on the things we've been giving our energy to that we need to let go of.

When we first enter this awareness, we have officially begun to wake up!

Asanas for Deepening

Practice uniting the body, mind, and spirit in celebration of our existence and of the vitality of the life force within us. Perform reclining twists, reclining hamstring stretch, seated yoga mudra, and tripod.

Reclining Twists

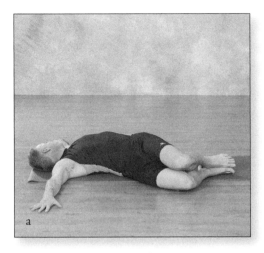

Knee over knee

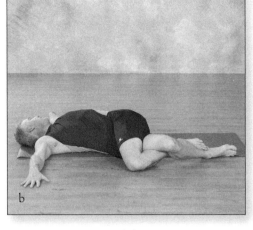

Eagle legs

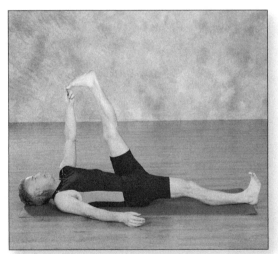

Reclining hamstring stretch

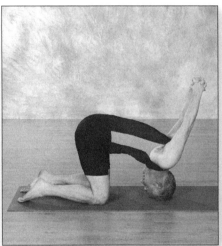

Seated yoga mudra

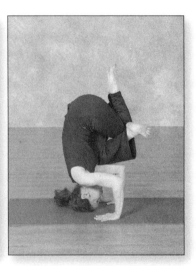

Tripod

Practice Off the Mat

Become aware of how important your attitude is in every aspect of your life. Attitude has the power to transform your experience of life itself. Live with intention.

Wise Words

If we are filled with toxins, tensions, and closed-down body parts, we won't have room for prana to flow.

Stay centered by accepting whatever you are doing.

Prana follows thought.

Feeling the Flame

Intention

To get a direct sensation of prana as it relates to life experience.

Approximate Length

3 to 5 minutes

Lesson

Today we will practice feeling a direct sensation of prana with a technique called "feeling the flame." This exercise explores emotions that bring pranic awareness of breath into our nadis, the subtle energy channels.

Let's begin by lying in shavasana. As you do this, recall the sensation of a very happy experience. This could be the feeling of falling in love, the birth of a child, or a fabulous vacation.

As you see this experience in your mind's eye, inhale the experience and begin to spread your arms slowly. Visualize your breath expanding from your heart center. This is an expanding flame that moves your arms effortlessly up toward your head. As your inner flame expands, your happy feeling expands with it.

Let the warm flames of happiness spread from the center of your heart, reaching out to the tips of your fingers and up to your head. As you exhale, feel it move down your legs into your toes.

Do this three to five more times. Go slowly and rhythmically. As you open, your body fills with breath awareness and happiness.

Please note: For many, the thought of warmth brings about body heat. Prana follows thought; be prepared to cool down!

Asanas for Deepening

With any asana, establish pranic intention. For instance, in parshvottanasana (angle), feel the pranic energy from the pelvic floor. In virabhadrasana I (warrior I), sense the pranic energy running from the back heel all the way up to the fingertips. In a seated forward bend such as paschimottanasana (posterior stretch), reach for your legs, ankles, or toes as if you were reaching for someone or something you love.

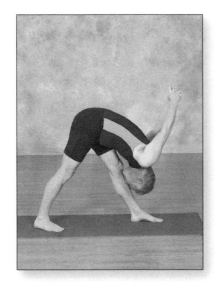

Parshvottanasana

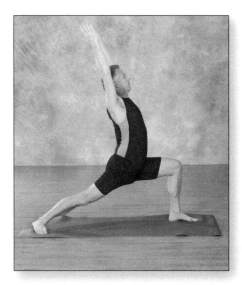

Virabhadrasana I

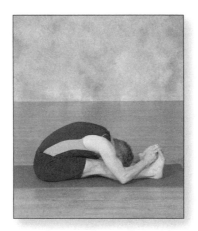

Paschimottanasana

Practice Off the Mat

Whenever you need to tap into the emotional power of your prana, you can get an instant vacation through creative visualization. Close your eyes and, in your mind's eye, see yourself on a sandy beach, in a cabin in the woods, or in the moment you first fell in love.

Wise Words

During asana, focus more on what you are doing with your prana than on your muscles and bones. What happens to the breath when a posture is easy for you? What about when a posture is difficult? What happens in your mind?

When you are in a posture, imagine the muscles in a favorite color, texture, or emotion. Then change the color, texture, or emotion and note how that affects your practice.

Prana and the Focused Mind

Intention

To understand how the mind affects prana.

Approximate Length

2 minutes

Lesson

Prana, or life force, is the vital energy of the universe. The human body exists by the same prana that sustains every living thing around us, just as the ocean is represented by a single drop.

Prana can be increased and decreased at will, and it can be moved here and there where we may need it. The process of learning postures and breathing techniques and of practicing meditation teaches us how to consciously control and move prana.

When we deal with circumstances such as managing stress, we can lose life force. .For instance, if we're worried about 10 different things, we may have prana bursting out of us in 10 different directions. Or if you are angry with someone or something, you are giving some of your available prana, your precious life force , to that person or situation. This loss of prana is draining to your energy and toxic to your system.

Learning to detach from negative situations is vital for keeping prana flowing. When we work with pranic intelligence, we work with and through stress, negative situations, and behaviors to create a calm, mindful mind.

Asanas for Deepening

Our asana practice gives us a system for identifying when, where, and how we are losing or blocking off energy. As you move through your postures, begin to notice where you are tight, weak, distracted, or uncomfortable. During ardha chandrasana (half moon), focus on the supporting leg and on moving energy into the pelvis and out into the limbs. Finish with kapotasana (pigeon), both the backbend (photo *a*) and resting (photo *b*) variations.

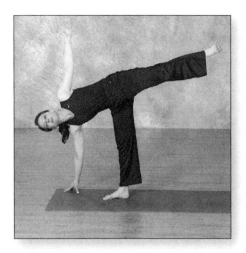

Ardha chandrasana

Kapotasana

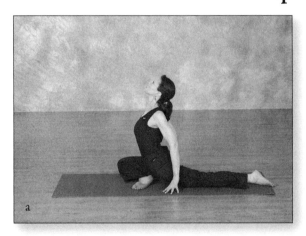

Backbend variation

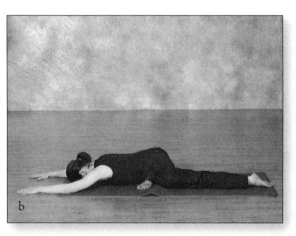

Resting variation

Practice Off the Mat

Embrace your prana. Limit your time and energy with people you find toxic. These could be coworkers, relatives, or even friends you need to distance yourself from.

Practice bhastrika breath (bellows) whenever you need a quick energy boost. Try three rounds of 11 breaths, drawing air in and out of the lungs very quickly. Bhastrika builds mastery of the energy flow in the body, energizing every cell and awakening serpent power (kundalini).

Wise Words

Mindful practice helps us remember that we can't tune into asana and be absorbed in a personal drama at the same time.

After holding postures such as seated twist, remember to feel the increased flow of energy through the spine.

Storing Prana

Intention

To learn how to store prana.

Approximate Length

5 to 7 minutes with prana-generating exercise

Lesson

Most of us begin practicing yoga to experience its physical benefits. But we stay because we begin to feel the esoteric benefits, many of which come from yoga's pranic power.

Prana is interwoven within the philosophy of hatha yoga and should be understood and acclimated within our yoga practices. To illustrate this point, consider that in ordinary breathing, we absorb an adequate supply of prana. Through controlled and regulated breathing exercises, however, we can elicit a greater supply so that we can store and use prana when we need it. We can then stockpile prana just as a storage battery can store electricity.

Today we'll work with a breathing exercise that stores prana in the solar plexus, the body's central prana storehouse—as well as the place that radiates strength and energy to all parts of the body.

Please lie down in shavasana. Bring your hands to the solar plexus and breathe rhythmically. After the rhythm is established, visualize how each inhalation draws in an expansive supply of prana, or vital energy, from the universal supply. This prana is taken in by the nervous system and is stored in the solar plexus.

On each exhalation, feel how each breath radiates strength and energy to all parts of the body. Imagine how the vital energy is distributed to every organ, every muscle, every bone, every vein, and every cell, from the top of your head to the soles of your feet. Feel it invigorating, strengthening, stimulating, and recharging every nerve center as it sends energy, power, and strength through every layer of consciousness.

Envision prana rushing in, coming in through the lungs and flowing into the solar plexus. Then exhale and savor the life force being sent to all parts of the body, out to the fingertips and down to the toes.

Asanas for Deepening

Agni sara (fanning) fans the flame of the solar plexus and distributes life force. It helps open and work the abdominal muscles, intestines, ovaries, fallopian tubes, uterus, spleen, gall bladder, kidneys, diaphragm, and lower back. From a standing position, bend forward and rest your hands just above your knees. Exhale completely and pull your belly back toward the spine (photo *a*). Without inhaling, let the belly drop, pull it back again, let it drop, and pull it back again (photo *b*). Repeat this process until you need to inhale. Repeat two or three times and feel the heat.

Perform navasana (boat) with the arms extended. This creates strength in the solar plexus.

Kapotasana (pigeon) with the foot to the elbow stretches the solar plexus and opens the hips.

Agni Sara

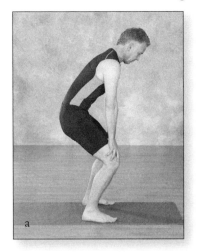

Belly pulled back

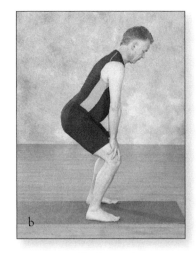

Belly dropped

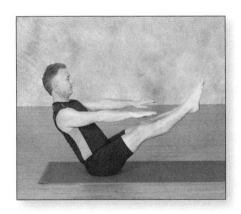

Navasana

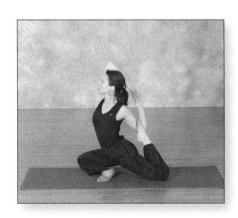

Kapotasana

Practice Off the Mat

Smile at any time during the day—do it now—and notice the calming effect on the body and heart center.

Look outside. Contemplate how nature is never at rest. From the smallest blade of grass to the world's largest ocean, everything is alive with pranic vibration.

Wise Words

Use intention. Do you want to stretch the hamstrings, calm an anxious mind, or make a decision? As you consciously inhale, allow universal energy to spread throughout the body. Make a mental picture of what you want to produce.

Sense the subtleties of breath. Sense the nadis being cleansed. Sense prana flowing through them.

Chapter 6
Pranayama

Each morning we are born again. What we do today is what matters most.

—Buddha

Our hatha yoga practices are designed to help unclog the nadis, the body's subtle energy channels, so that prana can flow freely and so that we can direct it toward more spiritual endeavors.

Pranayama, the fourth of the eight-limbed path of Raja yoga, is also referred to as "the last of the external limbs." Sometimes taught separately from postures, or neglectfully not at all, asana practice helps prepare us for more advanced breathing exercises by reducing body tension, opening up the breathing anatomy, and bringing awareness to the flow of breath.

Asana, united with pranayama and rightful living, directly supports the aspirant on his or her journey to enlightenment. On this glorious path of liberation, we visit all the transformational stops along the road.

What Is Pranayama?

Intention

To get a basic knowledge of the science and practice of pranayama and how it relates to the royal path.

Approximate Length

2 minutes

Pranayama Practice After Relaxation

5 minutes

Lesson

Pranayama is the fourth limb of the eight-limbed royal path as taught by Patanjali. Many students know it as a variety of breathing practices.

The word *pranayama* is a combination of *prana,* or life force, and *yama,* which means control. The practice of pranayama is the use of breath to bring life force under control.

Pranayama is an instrument that helps us control the thought waves of the mind. When we control the breath and prana, we control the mind. Inhalation is the process of drawing universal energy into the body and bringing the spiritual cosmic breath into contact with the individual breath. Exhalation is the removal of toxins from the system, providing room for prana to exist and expand.

A regular pranayama practice keeps the nadis, the body's subtle energy channels, in good health and prevents their decay.

Additionally, the physical practice of pranayama increases lung capacity. We breathe 23,000 times per day and use 4,500 gallons of air. With regular practice, we can learn to deepen the breath and utilize up to 6,000 gallons of air a day.

Today after relaxation, we'll have a short pranayama practice using anuloma krama. This breath is a segmented inhalation that fills the torso with prana and expands lung capacity.

Asanas for Deepening

Any practice that prepares the body for pranayama will stretch and strengthen the supporting anatomy around the lungs and diaphragm.

For thread the needle, get on your hands and knees. Thread the right arm behind the left arm and draw the right shoulder blade to the ground. Twist to the left. Repeat on the opposite side.

For twisting triangle, place one hand on the ankle or ground, or on a block in between the feet, and raise the other arm. Twist to the side of the raised arm. Repeat on the opposite side.

Ustrasana (camel) opens the front of the body.

During sarvangasana (shoulderstand), blood circulation is increased around the neck and chest, providing treatment for bronchitis, asthma, breathlessness, and throat ailments.

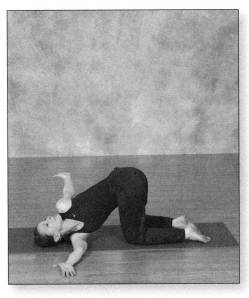

Thread the needle

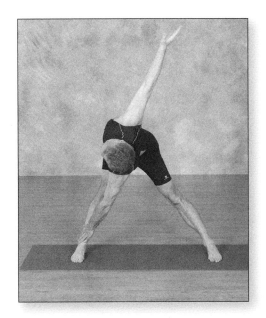

Twisting triangle

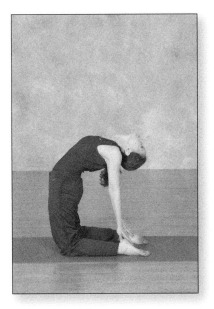

Ustrasana

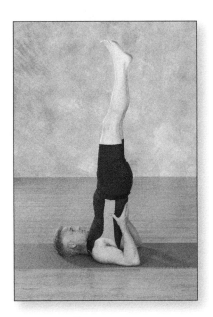

Sarvangasana

Anuloma krama. Use this segmented inhalation routine after relaxation.

1. Exhale deeply and fully.
2. Inhale the first third of breath in two to four seconds, expanding from pubic bone to navel center. Pause.
3. Inhale the second third of breath in two to four seconds, expanding from navel center to heart center. Pause.
4. Inhale the last third of breath in two to four seconds, expanding from sternum to throat center. Pause.
5. Exhale slowly and fully.
6. Repeat for five more breaths.

Note: As you inhale, visualize your torso as a tall glass. Each breath fills the glass with water until it's filled to the top. Exhale and pour out all the water.

Practice Off the Mat

In any situation, you have a choice to become the ego self-identity or an enlightened being. You have the choice to be uptight and hardened or relaxed and adaptable.

Wise Words

Keep the brain receptive and observant.

Tune the ears into the vibrations of the exhalation and inhalation.

Open your pores and breathe as if the skin breathes.

If we breathe incorrectly, we cannot achieve optimal health.

Yoga practice helps the breath connect the brain to the heart, and consequently, the world outside to the world within.

Benefits of Pranayama

Intention

To discuss the physical, mental, and spiritual attributes of pranayama practice.

Approximate Length

2 minutes

Pranayama Practice After Relaxation

5 minutes

Lesson

Pranayama is the current that removes impurities from our bodies, minds, intellect, and ego. The practice of pranayama increases lung capacity, which benefits every system in the body. During normal inhalation, an average person takes in about 500 cubic centimeters of air. During deep inhalation, we take in about six times as much.

The practice of pranayama has countless benefits:

- It purifies the nadis, protects the internal organs and cells, and neutralizes lactic acid, which can cause fatigue.
- It relaxes the respiratory muscles of the neck.
- It relaxes the facial muscles. When the face is relaxed, the muscles release their grip on the eyes, ears, nose, tongue, and skin—the organs of perception—lessening the tension in the brain. Concentration, calmness, and confidence are then present.
- Because the breath is linked to mental and emotional energy, the practice of pranayama helps change a negative mental attitude to a positive one.
- Pranayama improves digestion, vitality, perception, and memory.

After relaxation, we'll have a pranayama practice that includes nadi shodhana and kapalabhati, the shining skull breath.

Asanas for Deepening

For chest beating, make loose fists with the hands and gently beat the upper chest, shoulders, rib cage, and side ribs.

During the cat stretch, feel the movement of breath through the spine.

In parshvakonasana (triangle II), stretch from fingertips to toes.

Move into dangling uttanasana (standing forward bend), feeling the torso swell and lift slightly with each inhale, then release on the exhale.

Finish with a backbend series—bhujangasana (cobra, photo *a*), shalabhasana (locust, photo *b*), and dhanurasana (bow, photo *c*)—to open the breathing passages.

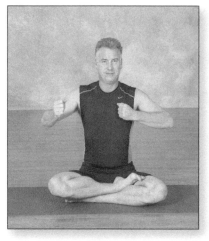

Chest beating

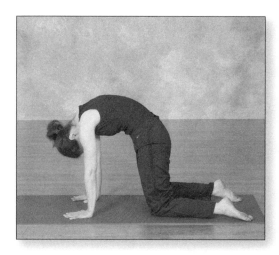

Cat stretch

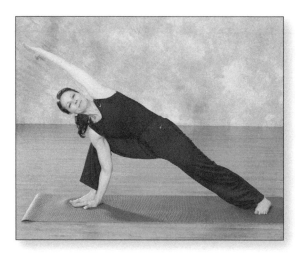

Parshvakonasana

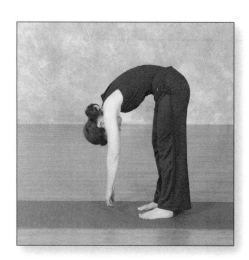

Dangling uttanasana

Backbend Series

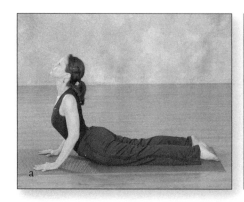

Bhujangasana

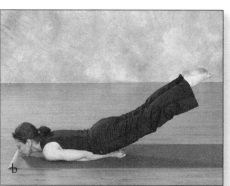

Shalabhasana

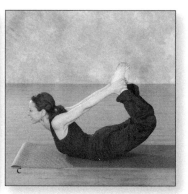

Dhanurasana

Recommended pranayama practice after relaxation:

1. One round of nadi shodhana (see page 29). Before you begin, check to see which nostril is active and which one is passive. Begin on the active side.
2. Eleven to 22 kapalabhati (shining skull) breaths. Kapalabhati is an invigorating, energizing, and purifying pranayama that cleanses the nasal passages and lungs, stimulates the brain, and energizes the body. To practice, force the exhalation deeply and quickly, pressing the diaphragm in and up, and follow with a normal inhalation.
3. One round of nadi shodhana. Begin with the passive nostril.

Practice Off the Mat

If you are feeling tired or dull, a longer inhalation can be useful; if you need to calm down, a longer exhalation will relax you.

Wise Words

Pranayama is one of the surest ways to attain mastery over the modifications of the mind, making it one-pointed (focused) and turning it inward.

With every breath, experience the newness of the now.

To be a yogi is to have the wisdom to remove anything that stifles your consciousness and makes you suffer.

Invite your mind to breathe into every part of the body.

Working With Ha and Tha

Intention

To learn how to balance the lunar and solar manifestations of the body and mind.

Approximate Length

5 minutes

Lesson

The essential practice of hatha yoga is to balance ha and tha, the solar and lunar currents that represent the dual nature of man: the sun and the moon, male and female, hot and cold, light and dark, mental and physical, right and left. This includes working with the two major nadis that manage our experience of the world: ida, the current that ends in the left nostril, and pingala, the current that ends in the right nostril.

When we become aware of nostril dominance, as we do in the practice of nadi shodhana, we realize that most of the time, one nostril flows more freely than the other. But when both nostrils are open, the central current, sushumna, is active. This is considered the most important nadi in the body.

The sushumna channel or conduit is the pathway to enlightenment through which awakened energy rises all the way from the core to the crown chakra, creating a state of balanced energy. This open pathway has been called "the way to liberation."

Pranayama exercises increase the capacity of the pranic body and mind so that we can manage the dual nature of the world and move back to equilibrium. This is the essence of balancing ha and tha.

Today we'll begin practice by working with ida and pingala. Get into a comfortable sitting position, with your head, neck, and trunk in alignment. Soften the belly and feel it naturally move with the breath. Now bring your attention to the sensation of breath in the active nostril. Focus on the breath as if it's flowing only through the active side. If thoughts outside of this practice come into your mind, let them go.

Now move your attention to the passive nostril. Feel the touch of breath and focus there without letting the mind wander. Stay here a bit longer than on the active side, and see if your focused intention opens the passive side.

Finally, direct your breath into both nostrils. Inhale from the nostrils inward to the crown of the head. Exhale from the crown to the nostrils. Let your mind relax as you breathe back and forth between these two points.

Asanas for Deepening

Multiply the benefits of your practice by using your full attention.

In malasana (squat), practice 11 bhastrika breaths (bellows breath). You will feel a subtle shift in energy in the nostrils when the pranic field is clear.

Finish with padmasana (lotus or half lotus).

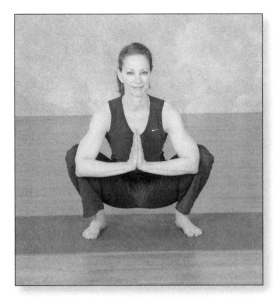

Malasana

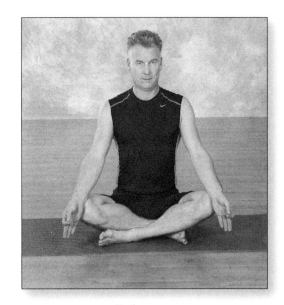

Padmasana

Alternate nostril with retention. Practice this exercise after two or three rounds of nadi shodhana and 11 to 22 bhastrika breaths. This is a powerful technique that rapidly alternates the flow of the breath from right to left. Begin in a seated position.

1. Fold the forearms into the belly.
2. Exhale and fold forward over your arms, bringing your face toward the floor.
3. Inhale deeply and retain the breath as long as comfortable, keeping the spine long. Return to an upright, sitting position.
4. Tuck in the chin, close the active nostril, and exhale forcefully through the passive nostril.
5. Inhale through both nostrils, close the passive nostril, and exhale forcefully through the active side. Repeat this exercise until both sides are flowing freely.

Caution: These techniques should not be practiced by anyone with high blood pressure or chronic problems in the eyes, nasal passages, or ears. If you feel dizzy or lightheaded, please stop.

Practice Off the Mat

Sustaining a balanced ha and tha can be a helpful approach to your day. For instance, if you need to do quiet work on the computer and you feel over-activity in the right nostril, try opening the left. Bring your awareness to the left, or try a few rounds of nadi shodhana with emphasis on the left channel in order to activate the right brain. Alternately, if you need to meet with clients, make a presentation, keep a social engagement, or anytime you require balanced external left-brain energy, activate the right nostril.

Wise Words

The place between ha and tha is where change happens. This is the place of balance and harmony.

Tension restricts the flow of life force.

Positive results from asana practice can come only from the absence of tension.

When you've reached your edge, don't go beyond it. Instead pause and breathe there so that you can feel the hot and the cold, the good and the bad, the sharp and the soft. Attempt to find the middle ground between ha and tha.

Pranayama Practice for the Immune System

Intention

To integrate into a traditional asana practice those pranayama practices that enhance the immune system.

Approximate Length

60 minutes with asana and pranayama practice

Lesson

Most of us get a cold or the flu once or twice a year. But if you're constantly sick, it could be a sign of an exhausted or compromised immune system.

The chakra most related to the immune system is manipura chakra, which is located at the navel center. This chakra is linked to the adrenal glands, which can be overworked during times of undue stress on the body and mind. If the adrenals are overworked, the immune system will be weakened.

To boost your immune system, include some asanas that work manipura chakra along with agni sara pranayama and two-to-one breathing. Drink 8 to 10 glasses of water a day and eat a diet rich in fiber in order to help the flow of food and toxins through the intestines. Include vitamin C and zinc in your daily supplement, and get plenty of sleep.

Asanas for Deepening

Immune system booster. The routine that follows will work manipura chakra and provide a boost to the immune system. Finish with shavasana. Always follow asana practice with relaxation for 5 to 10 minutes.

1. Surya namaskara (sun salutation) (see pages 58-59), one to three times
2. Agni sara (see page 85), three to five rounds
3. Fire series (leg lifts), one to six variations
4. Dhanurasana (bow) to balance agni (internal fire), two to three times holding for five breaths, followed with balasana (child's pose)
5. Paschimottanasana (posterior stretch) to eliminate accumulated toxins, boost the immune system, and improve circulation. Hold the pose for three to five breaths, and repeat six times. Practice deep exhalations as you fold into the pose.
6. Twists, such as easy twist or marichyasana, to help the cleansing process, one to three times each side.
7. Sarvangasana (shoulderstand) to soothe the nerves and help relieve hypertension and insomnia. It also stimulates the thyroid gland. Maintain the pose for 5 to 10 breaths, or longer if comfort allows.
8. Two-to-one breathing for two to three minutes
9. Shavasana

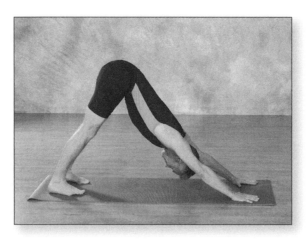

Surya namaskara

Agni Sara

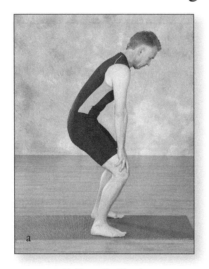

Belly pulled back

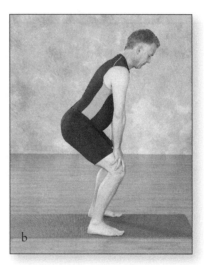

Belly dropped

Fire Series

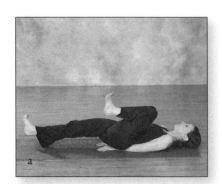

Bicycling

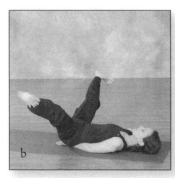

Spread-leg stretch

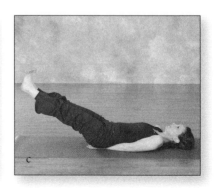

Double-leg lifts

Dhanurasana and Balasana

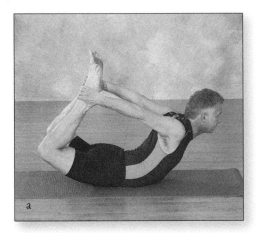

Dhanurasana

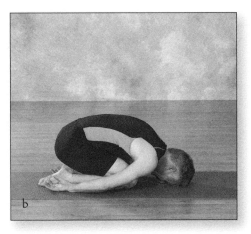

Balasana

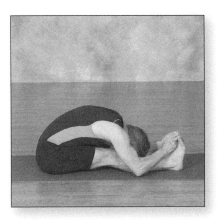

Paschimottanasana

Seated Twists

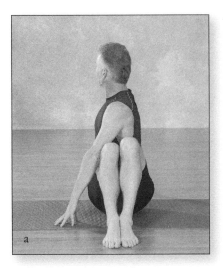

Easy twist

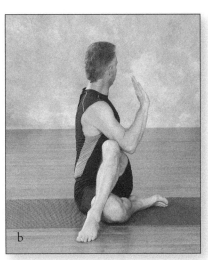

Marichyasana

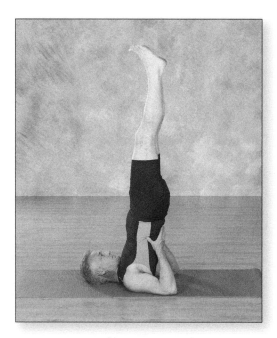

Sarvangasana

Practice Off the Mat

Spend time outside in the cold weather. During the winter months, most of us spend 90 percent of our time indoors, inhaling filtered air and other people's germs. Dedicate some time outdoors, breathe the fresh air, and allow the cold air to stimulate the thyroid gland.

Nurture your emotional being. Every few months, take a day off to simply nurture your being. Spend time with friends, indulge in a massage, or go to a workshop.

Sleep. A substantial factor in your overall well-being and balance is a full night's sleep. Your body needs time to heal and cleanse from its daily activities. In addition, sleep is linked to balanced hormone levels (including the stress hormone cortisol), weight management, and clear thinking.

Wise Words

More oxygen in your system gives the immune system more ammunition to fight off germs—another reason to breathe with awareness.

Practice the now, riding (instead of fighting) with the rhythm of your life as it is. When you're content, you're far less likely to become run down and sick.

Chapter 7
Yamas

On life's journey, faith is nourishment, virtuous deeds are a shelter, wisdom is the light by day, and right mindfulness is the protection by night. If a man lives a pure life, nothing can destroy him.

—**Buddha**

So much more than a physical discipline, yoga is a path to liberation. It is rich in an ancient philosophy that is as relevant today as it was thousands of years ago. As codified by the Hindu sage Patanjali, the yamas is the first limb of Raja yoga's eight-limbed path, which is comprised of five moral disciplines and restraints. Once processed, we find that each of the yamas apply to our daily lives. For now, consider each sacred value carefully as it relates to work, play, emotions, thinking, social interaction, and even the yoga we take to the mat.

Yamas: Moral Disciplines and Restraints

Ahimsa—Nonharming, nonviolence
Be gentle to yourself and to all creation. This includes refraining not only from physical violence but also from criticism and judgment.

Satya—Truthfulness
Avoid all falsehood and fabrication.

Asteya—Nonstealing
Do not take or covet what belongs to someone else, whether it's credit for someone's idea or physical objects.

Brahmacharya—Moderation in all things
Avoid excess in all areas of life.

Aparigraha—Nonpossessiveness
Abstain from greediness, hoarding, or possessing beyond one's needs.

Yama 1: Ahimsa

Intention

To teach nonviolence to yourself and others; to introduce the first of the five restraints.

Approximate Length

2 minutes

Lesson

The five yamas—the first step on the eight-fold path of Raja yoga—are restraints for cultivating happiness and self-confidence for a better inner and outer world. The first of these is ahimsa. Ahimsa refers to the practice of nonviolence. The yogis believe that there is no higher virtue than to do no harm.

Violence isn't limited to killing or hurting another person or animal. It can take many other forms, such as selfishness, anger, or negative words. The practice of ahimsa begins within. To paraphrase an ancient Taoist proverb, "If there is to be peace in the world, there must be peace between neighbors. If there is to be peace between neighbors, there must be peace in your heart."

Self-awareness is an important step for seeing how violence plays out in our existence, from the most subtle examples, such as self-criticism, to the most obvious manifestations, such as war.

Today's practice focuses on ahimsa in action and includes the application of patience, compassion, and love. Let's set our intention on inviting peace and stillness into our individual actions of body and spirit, and let's make a commitment to practice asana with ahimsa.

Asanas for Deepening

Be kind to yourself. Listen to your edges. Balance working with challenge and effort without working toward pain. Smile. Take pleasure in the posture. Enjoy what the message of the posture means to your practice of nonviolence.

Begin with standing yoga mudra. Let the weight of the arms open the back muscles. Feel your ribs sliding off your pelvis and the hamstrings and shoulders opening. Release the weight of the world.

During resting kapotasana (pigeon), remember to never force the openings.

From boat position (Navasana), grab your big toes with your first two fingers and gently press against the hamstrings, keeping the spine long and lifted.

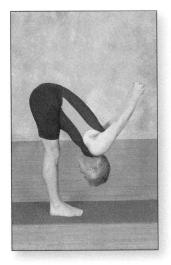

Standing yoga mudra

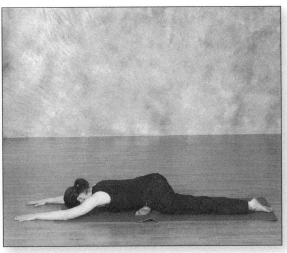

Resting kapotasana

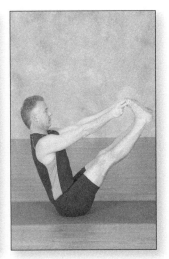

Navasana

Practice Off the Mat

Notice when you do harm yourself. This could be self-criticism, angry words, even eating the wrong foods. Then forgive yourself and rest in the awareness of knowing that ahimsa can be your guiding light of self-love.

Wise Words

Ahimsa comes from an awareness of action and thought, the same insight we practice in asana.

Ahimsa can be most challenging when we apply it to ourselves.

A careful and restrained use of force is sometimes necessary for preventing even greater violence. It's said that in one of his past lives, Buddha killed a man who was about to murder 500 others.

Asana practice is a powerful tool for liberating harmful emotions locked in the body's tissues.

Yama 2: Satya

Intention

To study yogic truth as defined by Patanjali.

Approximate Length

4 minutes

Lesson

In Patanjali's *Yoga Sutras*, Satya, or truthfulness, is identified as the second yama, or restraint, on the path of yoga.

What is truth? It seems that we each have a personal version of truth and what it means to us.. For instance, if three people witness a car accident, each person may have a different account of the same accident. We refer to this as *subjective* truth.

Truth is more than just not telling lies. The guiding principle in adhering to satya is to remove what the yogis refer to as "the veil of self-deception." By removing this veil, satya also translates as avoidance of distortion, embellishment, or *any* fabrication of truth.

Look at your life. Do you put your worries, anxieties, and fears into the things people say to you? Or do you listen without attaching to past conversations you may have had with that person? How truthful are you to yourself? Do you often embellish or exaggerate?

You may want to consider how the yamas help you formulate your daily life. Take a look at the first yama, nonharming. What happens when your best friend who has just spent a week shopping for the perfect dress buys it and asks you whether you like it? You feel the dress is not attractive on your friend. Do you tell her this? Our yoga philosophy suggests that if truthfulness brings more harm than good, our choice is to remain silent.

Like everything in our lives, we must weigh and balance thoughts, speech, and action in order to achieve a harmonious existence.

Today, notice the truth in your practice. Do you tell yourself that you can't do a pose even if you've never tried it? Do you tell yourself that a posture doesn't cause pain when it does?

Practice satya, working with honesty. To experience the liberating effects of asana, we listen carefully to our inner voice and discover that truthfulness is a remarkable tool for purifying our energies.

Asanas for Deepening

Keep honesty present in your practice. Ask yourself meaningful questions. Is the truth that your mind is wandering? Is the truth that you feel anxiety in a pose? Notice how prana is enhanced or cut off by a change in mental attitude.

During vrikshasana (tree), relax into holding your balance as you observe the interplay between your outer body and your will and ego.

While in virasana (hero), be alert to the truth of your skeletal system, including your ankles, feet, knees, thighs, and pelvic bones. Feel your weight sink toward the floor.

In janu shirshasana (head to knee), notice your mind's physical demand that suggests you should be where you're not naturally ready to be.

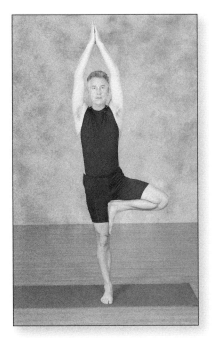

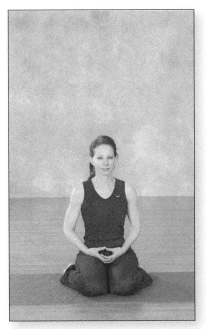

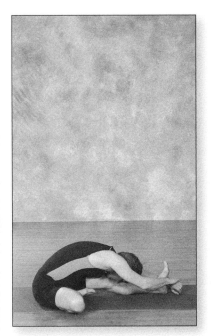

| Vrikshasana | Virasana | Janu shirshasana |

Practice Off the Mat

Sharpen your listening skills. Can other people's words obscure our own truth?

When my children were young, an older friend told me to cherish every moment with them; they would soon grow up and start their own families. Was she suggesting that I was asleep at the maternal wheel? Did I not appreciate my children? Or was I simply diluting her words with my defenses? When I listened with satya, I really heard what she was saying—to simply enjoy this time in my life. True listening allows us to surrender to another person's words without putting our own opinionated energy into them.

How often have you projected your own truths into someone else's words?

Wise Words

When body and mind are in sync, truth rises to the top.

Take time to listen for inner truth.

Telling the truth has little meaning until we first remove the veil of illusion.

As awareness expands, our perception becomes clearer, and we come closer to the truth, seeing life as it is in each moment.

Yama 3: Asteya

Intention

To define and explain the concept of Patanjali's asteya.

Approximate Length

2 minutes

Lesson

The third yama, or restraint, is asteya, the yama of nonstealing in the broadest sense of the word. Let me give you an example.

Carolyn was copywriter for an advertising agency. She worked with an art director, named Brian, to create ad campaigns. One Monday morning, as Carolyn shuffled passed the agency staff and into her office, she overhead the office clamor: "We were robbed over the weekend!" "What did they take?" "How did they break in?" Abuzz with the news, the staff was shocked and frightened. As Carolyn sat at her desk to take a quick inventory of her belongings, her partner, Brian, who was known for his wit as well as for his designs, came into her office and screamed, "They stole all my ideas!"

Although Brian's whimsical remark made light of the tense situation, this is an accurate definition of how asteya works in our lives. Asteya means much more than just not taking what isn't ours. But it also refers to not taking credit for actions that aren't ours, not accepting too much change from a cashier, not being late and thus not, in a sense, stealing time from the person who is waiting for us, and, yes, not stealing ideas.

Think about the ways that asteya may relate to our asana practice. In yoga class, we often compare ourselves to others, and we want what others have, whether it's their flexibility, strength, body shape, or an advanced forward bend.

Sometimes, when the body cannot perform a finished pose, we might strain or injure ourselves. We are violating the first yama, nonharming, as well as the second yama, truthfulness. As a result, we begin to see how the yamas build on one another, creating a foundation for life.

Asanas for Deepening

Practice postures that are challenging, if not downright impossible for you. Treasure the fact that you can bend forward, although you may need to bend your knees.

Let go of the craving to do a pose in the way someone else does it. Pick a headstand, lunge variation, crow, lotus, or balance posture, such as eagle, that is out of reach today. Make each posture your own and appreciate what you can do.

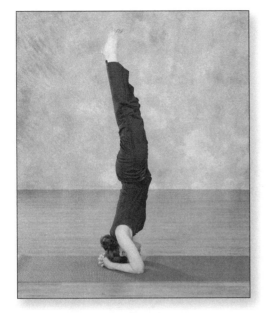

Headstand

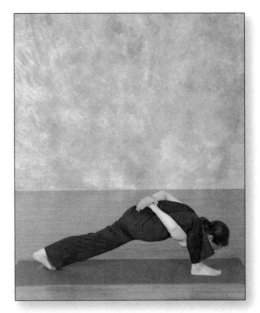

Runner's lunge with bound-arm balance

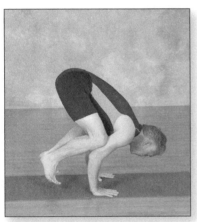

Crow

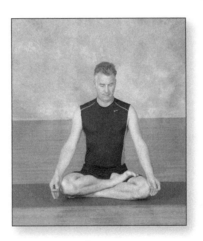

Lotus

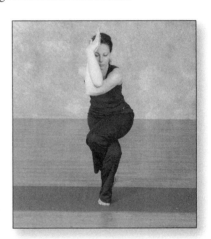

Eagle

Practice Off the Mat

Think about the ways you may steal without realizing it. Do you use office supplies for personal use? Do you use more natural resources than you need? Do you steal from nature?

Appreciate the things you have. When we look outside ourselves for more, we neglect the riches of our lives. Foster a sense of abundance in your life.

Wise Words

Don't steal energy from others. Just think of people who may drain you when they are around.

Be aware of taking up too much time with another person.

Cultivate a sense of completeness and self-sufficiency. Let go of cravings.

Yama 4: Brahmacharya

Intention

To introduce moderation in all aspects of living.

Approximate Length

3 minutes

Lesson

Imagine reaching for your third candy bar and hearing a voice in your head say, "Everything in moderation." That's the foundation of brahmacharya, moderation, the fourth yama.

Brahmacharya is commonly translated as celibacy, but this is not its only meaning. For everyday living, brahmacharya means to stop wasting one's energies. Patanjali's *Yoga Sutras* say, "When one is established in brahmacharya, or nonindulgence, one is endowed with inexhaustible energy."

Think about the things you indulge in—food, drink, caffeine, sleep, work, play, exercise, feeling depressed—the list goes on and on. As the saying goes, "Too much of anything is no longer good."

As yogis, we practice moment-to-moment awareness and inner clarity in order to expand on the bigger awareness of life. It's this process that allows us to respond to our true needs as we carefully listen to divine guidance and follow the path of moderation.

Brahmacharya on the yoga mat often teaches a new approach to our poses. We begin to explore the hows and whys of poses we indulge in and of those we resist. Many of us spend most of our practice doing poses that come easy, and we resist the ones that are challenging.

In today's practice, perform each pose as if you've never done it before—with a fresh, open mind and receptive body. Use a beginner's mind—there is no past, no future, only what is happening right now.

Listen and trust the voice within that always seeks balance, harmony, and peace in every movement and moment. As you let go of the bonds of past pleasures and pains, you might discover hidden abilities, new energies, and playfulness in your practice.

Asanas for Deepening

Practice any variation of surya namaskara (sun salutation, see pages 58-59) with respect for divine light above and within. Ask your inner spark what would feel right. Where is the brahmacharya within my surya namaskara? Brahmacharya is dedication to the perception, understanding, and awareness of the divinity within.

Practice deeply and honestly without spending too much energy on one pose or another. Coordinate holding postures with moving through them, lead by breath. Make sure to include poses that you normally resist, such as chaturanga or three-legged adho mukha shvanasana (three-legged downward dog).

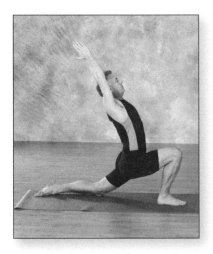

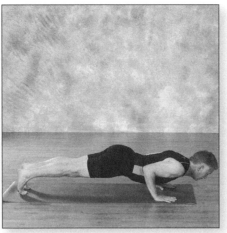

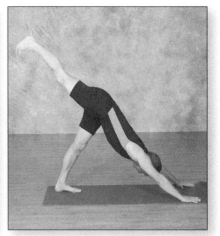

Surya namaskara   Chaturanga   Three-legged adho mukha shvanasana

Practice Off the Mat

Practice brahmacharya by meeting each moment with a fresh and new attitude. Experience the power and magic of the moment while going to work, hugging a loved one, or taking a deep breath.

Before taking that third piece of candy or drink, before sleeping too long or too little, or before surrounding yourself with toxic people, remember the benefits and goals of "everything in moderation."

Most yoga masters argue against casual sex. You don't have to switch off your sexuality. Just make each sexual experience count. Involve awareness of the heart. Sexual satisfaction begins with an open heart, and it blossoms through awareness.

Wise Words

Do you eat in moderation, think in moderation, talk in moderation, and do all activities in moderation?

Work toward an awareness of both energy and balance in order to avoid an emotional seesaw that can create overindulgence.

When our inner and outer lives are balanced, the mind becomes calm, our natural serenity flows, and we feel content with life.

Yama 5: Aparigraha

Intention

To learn to recognize greed within ourselves.

Approximate Length

2 minutes

Lesson

Aparigraha, nonpossessiveness, is the fifth yama, or yogic restraint. From a yogic perspective, possessiveness and greed are signs of a vacant search for happiness.

The desire to buy or accept more than is necessary clouds the mind and keeps us from understanding the deeper motivations and reasons of life.

So what is truly appropriate and necessary for us to be healthy, happy, and fulfilled? Ask yourself if you really need all the clothes, toys, or trinkets in your house. How much of it has become clutter?

The more possessions we have, the more attached we become to our things, the more our environments and minds become muddled and busy. You can see how easy it is to lose your perspective and connection to what is truly important in life.

Moreover, open your mind to the possibility that you may be attached to people such as your children, spouse, or friends. When this happens, there's no space to step back and simply appreciate the essence in those beings.

Likewise we can be possessive with our thoughts. We hold onto our ideas, our principles, and our ways of doing things. We become set in our ways. This a state of inflexibility that can transfer to our muscles and tissues.

The key to aparigraha is to learn to let go of attachment to possessions, people, thoughts, or ways of doing things.

Possessiveness often shows up in asana practice. Some people are attached to doing a perfect pose or to doing a pose a certain way. Others may be attached to old tensions or injuries or to a particular spot in the classroom.

Our challenge today is to detach emotionally from the posture, from the outcome, from what you think you are. Let go of your attachment to the practice or to the way you want it to be. This way, you can let the possibilities flourish.

Asanas for Deepening

When we attach emotionally to our strains and injuries, we block the natural flow of circulation in the muscles. When you feel tight, use breath awareness to create balance and space.

Let go of your expectations of how your body should perform or of how a pose should be practiced or taught. Only by letting go of ideas can we be open and receptive to the deeper experience of yoga. Each time we practice asana, we begin anew.

Begin and end your practice with shavasana (corpse pose). Practice total detachment. Lie down and let go of tension in your muscles and limbs. Let go of senses and thoughts so that you can be who you really are.

The rag doll stretch for the hamstrings and back teaches us about the power of letting go. Hang effortlessly with knees bent and tune into the vibrations originating in the spine. Feel them spread throughout the torso. Uttanasana is one of the ultimate surrender poses because *it* works *you*, not the other way around.

During gomukhasana (cow's face), relinquish your weight to the ground and spread out. Add the arms, but don't attach to "attaching" your fingers behind the back.

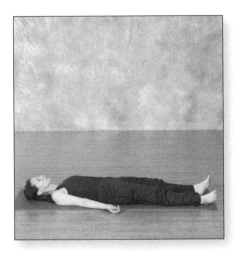

Shavasana

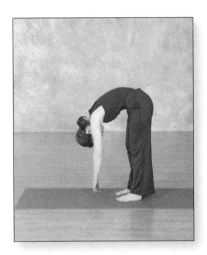

Rag doll

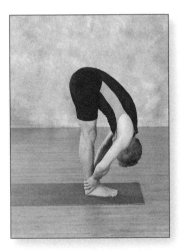

Uttanasana

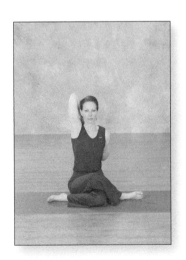

Gomukhasana

Practice Off the Mat

Do you have too much stuff? Do you tend to overeat? Are you so attached to your partner or child that you constantly worry about them? Are you envious of your neighbors? What happens when you don't get what you want?

When we let go of something, someone, or some expectation, we create space in our lives for new energies to come in. Loosen your mental grip on material possessions, and let go of the ego that is doing the gripping or grasping. Only when we let go of an idea of how life has to be can the moment naturally transpire.

Wise Words

The man who knows when enough is enough will always have enough.

The yoga practitioner who is well trained in the art of greedlessness is said to understand the deeper reason for life.

Don't cling to a person, place, or thing in the hope that it will bring you happiness. Clinging to that person, place, or thing will only bring you more clinging.

The possessions you acquire will never completely fulfill you.

Chapter 8
Niyamas

Even death is not to be feared by one who has lived wisely.

—Buddha

The second limb of Patanjali's eight-limbed path, the niyamas, offers practical advice for leading a healthier, happier life. The niyamas are five personal observances that direct the practitioner to exercise purity of mind in order to induce a natural state of joy and clarity. The observances are not intended to be strict and static; they are individualized, meant to be adapted as we adapt, ever-changing as we are.

Niyamas: Observances

Saucha—Purity

Keep your mind, heart, and body pure.

Santosha—Contentment

Accept life as it comes. Be satisfied with what is.

Tapas—Determined effort

Demonstrate the discipline or fire to bring about any kind of change.

Svadhyaya—Self-study

Study self, scriptures, and the internal states of consciousness.

Ishvara pranidhana—Surrender to the divine

Live with an awareness of the divine presence. Surrender ego-driven activities to divine energy.

Niyama 1: Saucha

Intention

To introduce the niyamas; to define saucha of body, mind, and spirit.

Approximate Length

1 to 2 minutes

Lesson

There are five niyamas, or observances, in yogic philosophy. The first one is saucha, which means self-purification.

Saucha is not only a foundation for physical health, it is also a way to cleanse the mind of negative emotions and thoughts.

As the mind works toward calmness and clarity, it becomes conscious of any toxins or disease in the body. Body and mind always work hand in hand. That is why fasting and cleansing techniques alone won't necessarily produce self-purification. If the mind is full of mental garbage, it must also come clean.

We'll focus our practice today on cleansing the body and the mind in order to allow more light and energy to flow. This practice allows us to focus on awakening our divine light within.

Asanas for Deepening

Uddiyana bandha (stomach lift) massages and tones the internal organs in the abdominal area as it relieves constipation, gas, indigestion, and liver trouble.

Malasana (squat) stimulates the digestive track and works the densest part of the body, the pelvis and legs, both of which are prone to retaining fat and water.

The change in gravity during sarvangasana (shoulderstand with knee twist) helps drain lymph as it stimulates digestion and elimination. In general, inversions, by the nature of being upside down, help loosen toxins in the body, and they encourage excess mucus to be excreted through the mouth and nose.

For simhasana (lion), begin by sitting on your heels. Come up on your knees and extend your arms out. Open your mouth and stretch the tongue out toward the chin. Exhale and roar, "Ahhhhh" like a lion. Repeat three times. Simhasana cleans the tongue and removes toxins from the throat and breath.

The squeeze-and-soak action of twisting postures, such as parivrtta parshvakonasana II (revolved triangle II) and marichyasana (seated twist), cleanses the organs. The squeezing forces out toxins and waste while the soaking releases fresh blood, bathing the cells with oxygen and nutrients.

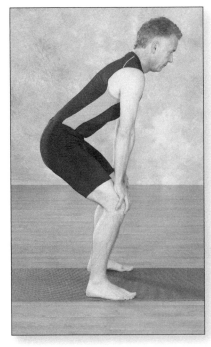

Uddiyana bandha

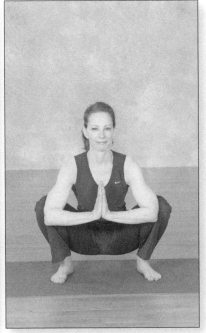

Malasana

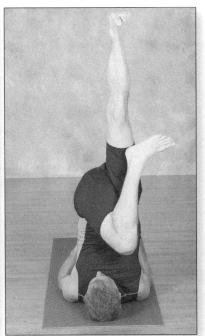

Sarvangasana with knee twist

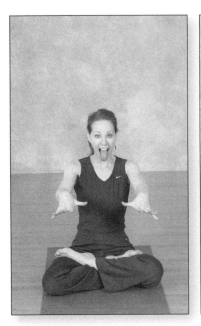

Simhasana

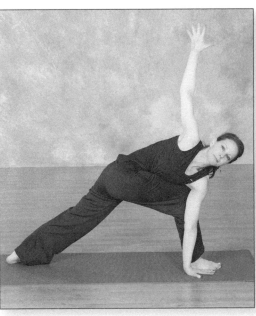

Parivrtta parshvakonasana II

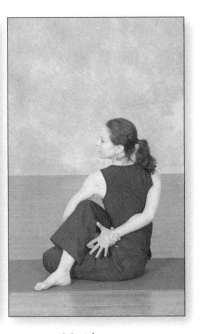

Marichyasana

Practice Off the Mat

For the mind to be clear, the body, as well as the surroundings of the body (home, office, practice space, yoga mat), must be clean.

Keep energy flowing within your environment. Don't let dirty dishes, laundry, unread mail, or garbage pile up.

An excellent method of cleansing the nasal passages is to use a neti pot. Fill the neti pot with a mild, lukewarm saltwater solution, then put the spout of the neti pot to one nostril, closing it off. Tilt the head to the side to allow the saltwater solution to pour from the closed nostril through the open one. Repeat on the opposite nostril. This removes mucus and buildup from the sinuses and nostrils, keeping the nasal area clear.

Bathe once a day, and move your bowels once a day, if possible. If the system is sluggish, toxins stay trapped in your body, keeping tension, anger, and slothfulness locked within the tissues. If your system is slow, practice deeper, longer-held twists, such as supine twists, before getting out of bed. Drink eight glasses of water a day, avoid white flours, and load up on fibrous foods.

Wise Words

The body, breath, and mind have an automatic cleansing process. The breath ebbs and flows, and thoughts enter and leave constantly. On every level, waste is released and replaced with energy and light.

From the perspective of Ayurveda—the sister science of yoga—the accumulation of internal waste is the primary cause of disease.

Niyama 2: Santosha

Intention

To recognize the significance of acceptance and choice as they relate to contentment in daily living.

Approximate Length

3 minutes

Lesson

Santosha, or contentment, is the second niyama, or observance, in yogic philosophy. We tend to think of contentment as the fulfillment of desires, but the yogis tell us that this kind of happiness is short-lived. As we learn from the yama aparigraha, or nonpossessiveness, desires create more desires and more cravings. Like a well that can never be filled, greed is a vacant search for happiness.

The yogic view of contentment develops from accepting whatever life brings us. Contentment is the mindfulness of living in the moment, something we naturally apply to asana.

There's a parable about two women who, from an outsider's perspective, seemed to live similar lives. Both were the same age, had the same-sized home, same-sized family, and same income level. The two women even looked alike. There was only one significant difference: One woman was satisfied with her life, while the other felt empty and frustrated. As we see from this parable, happiness—the feeling of contentment—is a choice.

Once you decide that what you have is all you need, contentment will always find a place in your heart.

Santosha requires a sense of inner acceptance, which begins when you stop comparing yourself with others. As long as there's comparison accompanied by judgment, there cannot be contentment.

Today in our asana practice, let's accept what we have. Let's accept what brought us here today. Let's accept our bodies, abilities, and limitations as they are right now. Enjoy the journey!

Asanas for Deepening

Personal practice will help you accept your body as it is and will allow you to lose your classroom competitive edge.

During trikonasana (triangle), witness the breath flowing into the awkward spaces. Stay in the pose and watch your body unfold through breath, time, and patience. If something feels disagreeable, stay unattached to the outcome and observe whether what you feel is pain, curious sensation, or emotional discomfort. Does santosha arise, even for a moment?

Setu bandha sarvangasana (bridge) allows us to open our heart, and thus our experience, to the truth and beauty of our inner and outer worlds. The posture keeps us from shutting out the reality of our needs, and it allows us to enjoy the sensation of the present. Let yourself be free of the past so that you can experience the gratification of the now.

In natarajasana (king dancer), feel the cause and effect, the ebb and flow, the strength and flexibility of the pose. Notice how prana moves you, creating more space in your field of energy. Conversely, does the breath struggle, thereby blocking energy flow, and shut you down? The choice is yours. Where are you resisting? On the other hand, where is there movement? Where is there a feeling of peace?

The anti-blues flow is a quick fix for the everyday blues. Practice moving from urdhva mukha shvanasana (updog, photo *a*) to adho mukha shvanasana (downdog, photo *b*) on the breath. Inhale into updog, exhale to downdog. Move in and out of these poses 6 to 20 times.

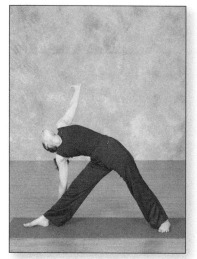
Trikonasana

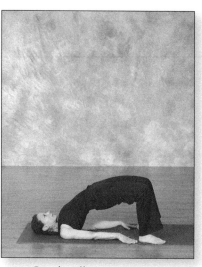
Setu bandha sarvangasana

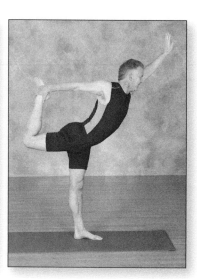
Natarajasana

Anti-Blues Flow

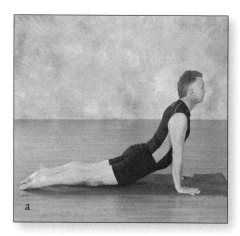
Urdhva mukha shvanasana

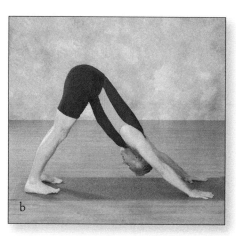
Adho mukha shvanasana

Practice Off the Mat

The purpose of contentment is to help us see that we're exactly where we're supposed to be right now. Know that there is something to learn from everything, everyone, and every experience.

Find the time to experience and enjoy the things that give you a happy feeling. Ask yourself how contentment shows up in your life. Do you find it while taking a walk in the woods, reading a good book, sipping a cup of coffee with a friend, or holding hands with someone you love?

Practice santosha each day by remembering the blessings you have in your life. There are thousands of extraordinary things around you if you choose to look at them that way.

Wise Words

Happiness is a way of travel, not a destination.

Contentment brings us into the moment, producing a sense of happiness into our lives right now.

Santosha means to free the mind of the mundane emptiness, the trivial irritations of life that take up too much of our spirit. When we can let go of daily technicalities, we see life in a larger context—with detachment and inner balance.

Accept what you have, and enjoy what you have. Only by acceptance can we find contentment.

Contentment allows us to know that whatever we are doing, we're making the right choice for ourselves.

Niyama 3: Tapas

Intention

To define tapas as the willingness to do whatever it takes to attain a necessary goal.

Approximate Length

2 minutes

Lesson

Tapas, the third of the niyamas, or yogic observances, is defined as the willingness to do whatever is necessary to reach a goal.

Tapas is about austerity, sacrifice, and discipline. It's defined as "heat" or "fire," and therefore tapas refers to the fire that brings about transformation. When we describe someone who is working hard at something, we say that they have a "fire in the belly."

According to the sages, fire that's created through yoga practice destroys pollution in one's consciousness and leads to the control of the body and senses. Therefore, there can be no yoga without tapas.

Consequently, in order to affect change on any level—whether it's to lose weight, change jobs, achieve hanumanasana (splits), or attain enlightenment—we must constantly commit to tapas.

A requirement of tapas is to cut through distractions and to bring our full attention to the present moment. To apply tapas, we might begin by observing the quality of mindfulness that we bring to an activity. How often do we focus 100 percent on something?

When we apply tapas to our asana practice, we can open up to a new level of discrimination. We don't practice mechanically, doing the same poses with the same intensity every day. Instead we practice mindfully, with determined effort, in order to affect change.

Asanas for Deepening

Be the pose. Exercise your awareness as you exercise your body. Put the effort in, and you'll get the change you need.

During the plank, visualize a flame at the navel center as you hold the pose. Expand the internal fire with your focus and breath. Notice the feeling of heat, strength, and power.

During parshvottanasana (side angle), keep your weight on the balls of the feet. Spread the shoulder blades and elongate the spine starting at the back of the skull. Move energy from the pelvic floor into the navel center. Inhale and bring vitality and life force into the whole body. Exhale and guide that force throughout your body.

Finish with the fire series of leg lifts. Keep the concentration on the navel center while continuing to fuel the fire of tapas. There are several variations of the fire series. Leg lifts can be practiced while on the elbows or, for more challenging classes, while lying on the back with the navel center pressed to the lumbar spine and the lumbar spine pressed to the ground. Lifts that can be included in this series include bicycle leg movements, leg circles, single- and double-leg lifts, horizontal and vertical scissors, and jathara parivartanasana (leg lifts with twist).

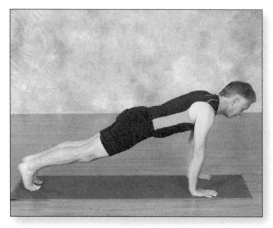

Plank

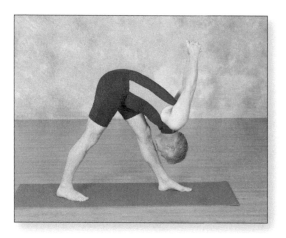

Parshvottanasana

Fire Series

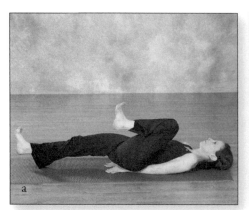

Bicycling

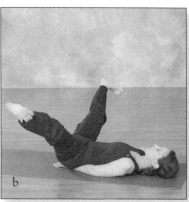

Leg circles

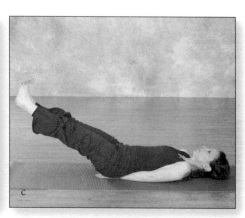

Double-leg lifts

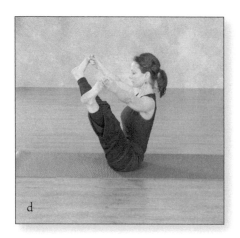

Navasana

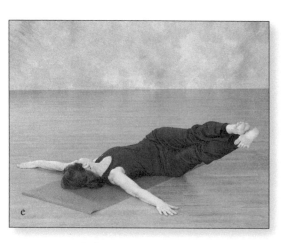

Jathara parivartanasana

Practice Off the Mat

Tapas may be summed up as, "Where there is a will, there is a way." If you often say to yourself, "I want to practice yoga daily, and I will find time for it," this will is the tapas.

Will yourself to make one small, positive change in your life every day. For instance, you may want to drink a glass of water every afternoon, call your mother, or simply commit to washing your dishes every night. Find what you need to will in your life, and commit yourself to the fire of tapas.

Wise Words

Sitting meditation is a disciplined practice during which physical heat is generated. The physical heat burns away the ego and thereby reveals the true inner spirit.

Tapas is stirred by the knowledge that life is a gift and by the desire to make the most of it.

Yoga is about being able to purify and undo anything that holds you down and makes you suffer.

Without self-discipline, one's actions, words, and thoughts become scattered, and prana becomes weakened.

Niyama 4: Svadhyaya

Intention

To define svadhyaya; to search out the meaning of spiritual concepts through self-study, questioning, and experience.

Approximate Length

2 minutes

Lesson

Today we're going to discuss the fourth niyama, or observance, svadhyaya, which means self-study or self-observation. The practice of self-study refers to both the understanding of the self through the study of sacred texts, as well as to the skill of self-observation, which leads to yoga or unification.

Svadhyaya is the effort to know the self—the inner self as well as the outer self—of universal consciousness.

One method of self-study is to study writings that inspire us to feel the presence of the inner spirit. We can then apply these inspirations to our lives so that they are meaningful to us.

In our asana practice, svadhyaya helps us observe moment-to-moment changes in our body and mind. How are you feeling in your body? Is your mind present? What subject matter draws your mind away? Applying svadhyaya to the yoga postures is a way of looking within and connecting to your inner truth.

Today as we practice and move and focus, go inside. Pause between your postures; listen and learn from them. Be honest about what you don't know or don't understand. Let yourself learn from the experience.

Asanas for Deepening

Practice self-study through breath awareness. Turn your attention inward and become aware of your breathing. Imagine and feel how the breath creates spaces in the abstract parts of the body and how it allows them to open and vibrate within. Feel the prana, the life force, activating every layer of consciousness.

Almost everyone has a definitive response to gomukhasana (cow's face). Do your fingertips reach each other? Are your hips opening for the first time? How can gravity help you release further?

During bhujangasana (cobra), observe how prana runs up the front of the spine and down the legs. Notice the chest opening, breath moving into the upper lungs. Relax in makarasana (crocodile) and feel the back tingle as your energy and mood shift.

Use upavistha konasana (seated angle) to gently expand your self-knowledge. Take yourself to your limit through astute awareness and through physical and mental adjustments. Study the pose without stepping back from or going over the edge. Challenge yourself to stay mindful.

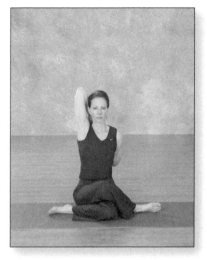

Gomukhasana

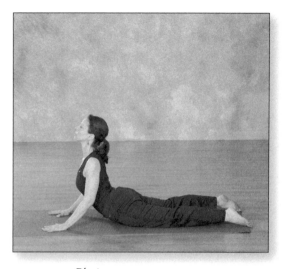

Bhujangasana

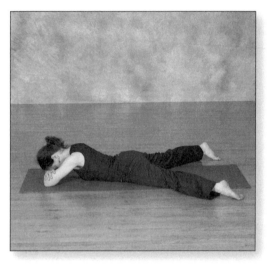

Makarasana

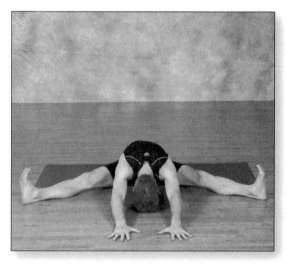

Upavistha konasana

Practice Off the Mat

Remind yourself to practice constant self-observation and self-study in daily living. Every movement is asana, every breath is pranayama, every thought is meditation. Before retiring each night, ask yourself, "What did I learn today?"

Wise Words

Svadhyaya gives you pause to breathe, relax, feel, and learn. Be open to receive and enjoy the spirit of exploration within you.

Study and practice go hand in hand. Acquire some useful yoga reference books and scriptures such as Patanjali's *Yoga Sutras*, *Hatha Yoga Pradipika*, and the *Bhagavad Gita*. As you study, discover how the concepts in these books change over time as you uncover the deeper meanings of life.

Niyama 5: Ishvara Pranidhana

Intention

To practice with faith and dedication to the divine energy of the universe.

Approximate Length

2 minutes

Lesson

The fifth niyama, or yogic observance, is ishvara pranidhana. This observance engages your relationship to the divine energy of the universe, and it honors a higher ideal or spiritual consciousness in your life.

When you surrender your ego-driven activities to divine spirit, doorways open for positive energy to flow into all areas of your life. According to the sages, by uniting your individual self with that of a higher divine principle—be it God, Buddha, Jesus, or nature itself—all egotism, trivialities, and selfishness are removed.

Every action we take can be done with significance, every word we speak can be spoken with meaning and truth, and every thought we have can be thought with clarity.

Today, take your practice within, find out the truth of who and what you are. Offer the fruits of yourself, your work, and your love to the divine spirit or spark within. Notice what a difference it makes when you surrender your ego and completely free yourself to something bigger than yourself.

Asanas for Deepening

When we practice asana with a sense of devotion to a higher purpose, it becomes a vehicle that permeates our lives. We relax and become more genuine and receptive in our practice.

Begin with namaste circles. Move the arms up over the head and out to the sides, with the palms connecting in namaste over the heart. Inhale and move the arms upward and outward (photo *a*). Exhale and move the hands to the heart (photo *b*). Feel the universal spirit within the heart center.

In tripod, rest the knees onto the shelf of the forearms. This posture helps to awaken the crown chakra, our connection to divine consciousness, which is located at the top of the head.

In standing squat, bring the hands in namaste over the heart. Feel the connectedness in the feet and legs. Bring both earth and heaven energy into the heart center.

Namaste Circles

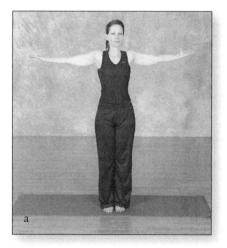

Inhale, move arms up and out

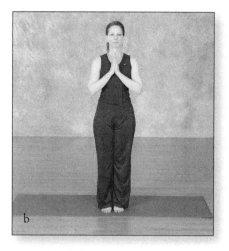

Exhale, bring hands to heart

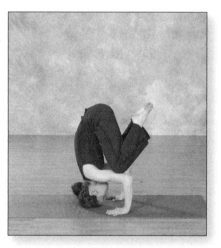

Tripod

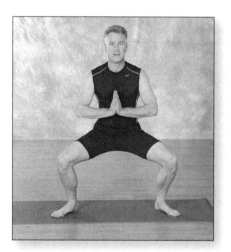

Standing squat

Practice Off the Mat

Meditate on what you do each day, who you talk to, where your mind goes, how your body moves. Start your meditation when you wake and continue it as you brush your teeth, eat your breakfast, go to work, and so on through the rest of your day. How does ishvara pranidhana weave into your daily activities?

Wise Words

The practice of ishvara pranidhana is a way of living in which you are always aware of the divinity of the supreme intelligence.

It is wonderfully illuminating to connect our small lives with the larger whole.

Practice having faith, dedication, and patience.

Surrender to the universe or to the divine, and ask for guidance.

Chapter 9
Emotions

What we think, we become.

—**Buddha**

When we awaken to the emotional side of yoga asana, we become more sensitized, perceptive, and responsive both on and off the mat. Ironically, the definition of yoga asana is a position that is both steady and comfortable, a place where one can feel completely present. From this silent backdrop, we watch the agitated mind. Practice then becomes a purifying method of listening to the inner workings of the mind and emotions.

The lessons in this chapter will help you recognize the emotions that arise during practice so that you can become more aware of them during your day. Don't criticize yourself if you find that negative emotions seem to lead the way. There's no place here for judgment. Just look, listen, and be aware.

Pay attention.

Emotional Effects of Asana

Intention

To present yoga's harmonizing effects on emotions.

Approximate Length

2 minutes

Lesson

Have you ever noticed the effect that your yoga practice has on your emotions? It's like a welcome sense of spaciousness, as though we've cleaned a room in our inner selves so that healing, along with light, come shining through.

Usually the positive emotions come to the surface: our sense of humor, patience, concentration. As we surrender and let go of frustrations, fear, and worry, we start to feel like our old selves again.

The flip side of this, of course, occurs when the negative emotions arise and stay with us. Naturally, if we're doing what we're supposed to be doing—cleansing and releasing—feeling our negative emotions is paramount to the process of renewal.

When this happens, give yourself space to feel what you're feeling. Instead of suppressing these emotions, realize that these feelings arose for a purpose. Then do your best to stay mindful of them, giving yourself enough room to eventually free these emotions from your spirit.

Our poses can strongly influence our emotional states. For instance, because of the expansive inhalation and opening of the chest, backbending, traditionally a stimulating practice, can elevate a low mood. Exhale-intensive poses such as forward bends tend to calm an agitated mind. In any balance practice, both inhale-oriented and exhale-oriented postures are executed in order to create equilibrium in the body and breath and to gain emotional harmony.

Today's practice will focus on restoring equipoise, empowering ourselves to release emotionally and to make positive changes in our layers of consciousness.

Asanas for Deepening

Sarvangasana (shoulderstand) or halasana (plow) help reverse energy blocks—inflexible thinking, stuck emotions, and feelings of sadness.

Balasana (child's pose) sends relaxing signals to both sympathetic and parasympathetic nervous systems.

Garudasana (eagle) offers relief to the scattered mind and works on the balance of the external and internal worlds.

Marichyasana (half seated twist) is one of yoga's greatest harmonizers because it both calms the mind and releases sluggishness in the body.

Janu shirshasana (head to knee) relieves feelings of anxiety, fearfulness, and stress. On each exhalation, let the torso sink further toward the legs.

Dhanurasana (bow) helps stimulate the inhale and arouses the adrenal glands.

Woodchopper assists in the emotional release of frustration and anger. While standing, lift your imaginary ax on your inhale, and with a forceful "Ha!" on the exhale, chop the imaginary wood between your legs.

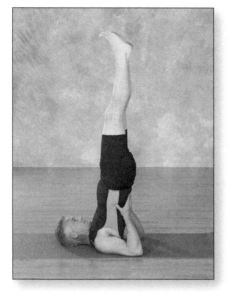

Sarvangasana

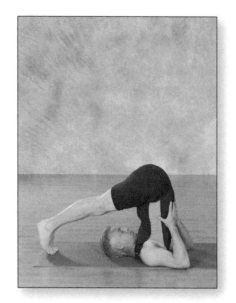

Halasana

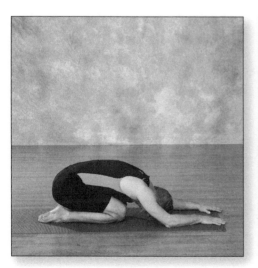

Balasana

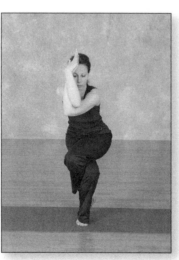

Garudasana

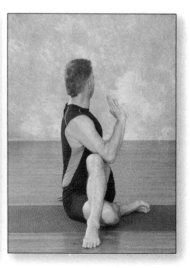

Marichyasana

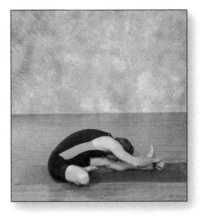

Janu shirshasana

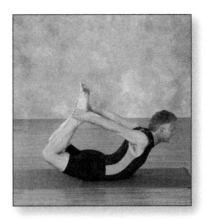

Dhanurasana

Woodchopper

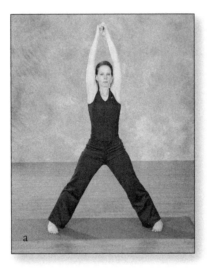

Arms above head

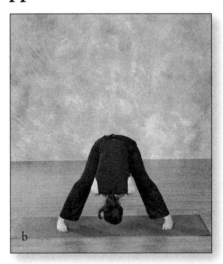

Arms between legs

Practice Off the Mat

Notice the situations that cause you to become tense. Are you an anxious driver, talker, or worker? When you cook or do the dishes, does your back feel strain? Whether the tension is in the shoulders, neck, back, or navel center, practice moment-to-moment body awareness. This will help you cleanse your negative emotions and trapped issues so that they don't find a permanent home in your body.

Wise Words

Following the path of yoga cuts through the roots of suffering.

Hatha yoga teaches us control of breath and control of body. Through awareness we learn concentration, control of our thought patterns, and emotional control. The serious yoga practitioner will cling less to life's negative matters, permitting the practice to have a leveling effect on the emotional body.

Frustration in the Body

Intention

To become aware of how the body manifests frustration.

Approximate Length

3 minutes

Lesson

When we feel frustrated, it generally means that we're not flowing with the experiences of our lives. Instead we're pushing away or resisting something. Frustration then collects in the body. Many of us feel it in the shoulders, neck, low back, and hips.

Problems in the shoulders represent irritability and resistance to change. Issues in the back can be related to a repression or restriction in your life, hurtful issues from the past, or the need to carry the weight of the world. Repressed anger creates tension in the neck as you force your feelings down your throat instead of saying what you want to say. You can literally experience a pain in the neck from something or someone who makes you angry. The hips are related to general frustration. Notice the person who often stands with her hands on her hips. This is a gesture of feeling frustrated and out of control.

Through a balanced asana practice, and particularly through the postures that work on these specific areas, many of our frustrations can be released. Let's set our intentions for today's practice on working out any frustration that manifests in any of these areas.

Please lie in shavasana. Breathe deeply into your belly, putting all of your awareness into the breath. Feel all the emotions of your respiratory system—the air in the nostrils, throat, and chest, the belly and chest rising. Feel the rib cage expanding to the front, to the sides beneath the armpits, and all the way into the lower back. Gently move your attention from your mental state to your breath so that you can more easily observe and step back from your emotions.

Asanas for Deepening

Reclining twist works on releasing frustration in the hips. Lie on your back. Stretch your arms out to the sides at shoulder height, palms down. Inhale and bend the left knee to your chest. Exhale and twist to your right side, releasing a deep audible sigh, "Ahhhh." Inhale and return to the back. Practice three times to each side. This twist is also helpful for relieving sciatica, headaches, and low-back stiffness.

There are several variations of neck stretches to practice: ear to shoulder (photo *a*), look over the shoulder (photo *b*), drop chin to chest (photo *c*), neck rolls.

Shoulder work can be done while seated or standing. Begin with arm circles (photo *a*). Hold a shoulder-width length of strap in front of you. Inhale and move your arms forward and up toward the sky. Exhale and bring your arms behind you, using the full range of motion in the shoulder joints.

Next move into arm pulls (photo *b*). Raise the left arm up, bringing the left arm alongside the left ear. Reach the right arm down and out, stretching through the fingers. Inhale and energize upward through the left arm. Exhale as you reach out your right arm and hand. Practice several breaths before alternating arms.

Finish the shoulder work with the collarbone stretch (photo *c*). Interlace your fingers behind you. Open the chest, bend the elbows, and bring the knuckles to the right side of the waist. Feel the left shoulder blade coming in toward the spine. Roll the shoulders back while squeezing the elbows together. Switch sides.

Cat stretch releases frustration in the back, pelvic floor, abdomen, and back of the neck.

Naukasana (boat) works on the acupressure points related to general bodily frustration, body aches, digestive problems, and fear. Lie on your abdomen with your chin on the floor. Stretch your arms straight out in front of you. Slowly and deeply inhale, lifting the arms, chest, head, and legs off the ground while arching the back. Hold for three to six breaths. Relax in child's pose.

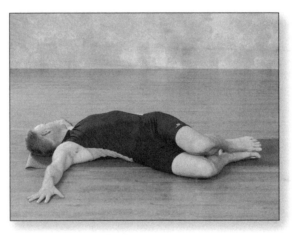

Reclining twist

Neck Stretches

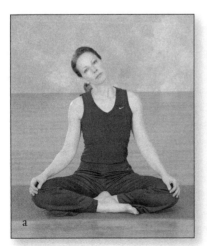

Ear to shoulder

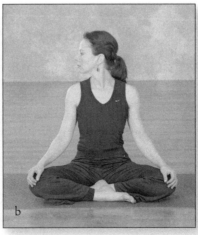

Look over shoulder

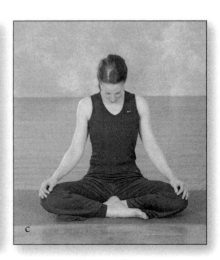

Chin to chest

Shoulder Work

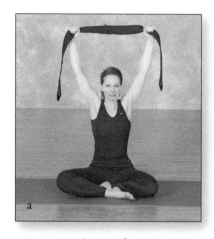

Arm circles

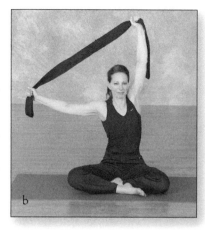

Arm pulls

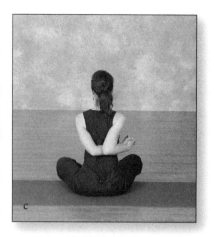

Collarbone stretch

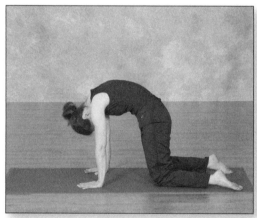

Cat stretch

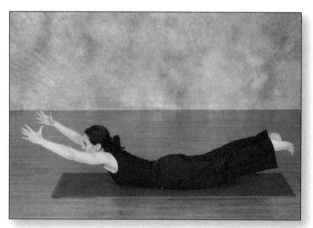

Naukasana

Practice Off the Mat

Body language has so much to do with how you express your emotions. Do you hunch your shoulders in an effort to protect or shield yourself? Do you often settle your hands on your hips? Notice your emotional frustration and then recognize how it manifests in your body.

Wise Words

The more we let go and release in all areas of our life, the more life unfolds itself to us.

With daily practice, patience, and faith, energy blocks will diminish, inviting health, healing, and life force into your being.

Each new breath is a new moment of life; the practice is to find the newness in each moment.

Embracing Change

Intention

To welcome change into our lives.

Approximate Length

1 minute

Lesson

Through the practice of yoga, we awaken to how life unfolds moment by moment. Things are constantly changing—the breath, your state of mind, the phases of the moon, the seasons. This can be both a profound revelation—life is like a flower that blooms continuously—and a harsh reminder that nothing lasts forever. Even your body will let you down in the end.

When we resist change, the ego will try to hold on to the body as it is. Consequently the body contracts and tenses, and the natural flow of energies slows down or may stop completely, creating blocks in the form of a tight hip or frozen shoulder. That's why until we accept the changes that occur from day to day and from year to year, and until we surrender to the natural course of existence, little progress can be made along the path of yoga.

Asana practice shows us how our bodies, minds, and the world around us are constantly changing. Today, through breath, patience, and a watchful eye, we'll honor our changes from movement to movement and embrace the reality of change.

Asanas for Deepening

From the first stretch of the morning to the more mindful and heated surya namaskara, we can feel and sense the immediate transformation in our bodies. Make sure you ground your awareness in the changes in breath, circulation (including body temperature), and muscle flexibility.

Psychologically, inverted yogic practices such as shirshasana (headstand, photo *a*), sarvangasana (shoulderstand, photo *b*), or halasana (plow, photo *c*) make us feel that the world is turned upside down. If we could get used to that feeling, we could adapt to change when it happens without warning.

Before taking the completed posture of parivrtta trikonasana (revolving triangle), twist from the waist, with the arms extending out to the sides (photo *a*), coming back to center several times until you sense the opening in the lower back and waist. Then take the full posture (photo *b*).

During ardha baddha padma paschimottanasana (half-bound lotus posterior stretch), as you exhale, stop when you feel the slightest resistance. Stay at this place until something changes, until you sense a new edge.

Inverted Postures

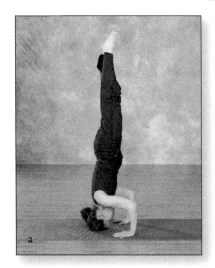

Shirshasana

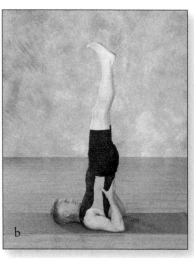

Sarvangasana

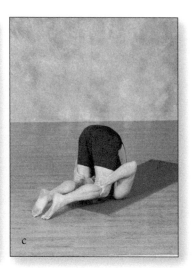

Halasana

Parivrtta Trikonasana

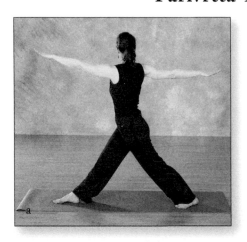

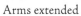

Arms extended

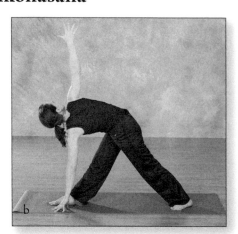

Full posture

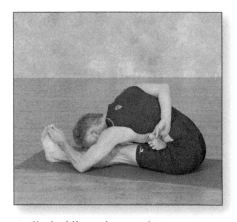

Ardha baddha padma paschimottanasana

Practice Off the Mat

Practice being open and receptive to change. Something as simple as changing your hairstyle or wearing different-colored clothing can give you a refreshing perspective on the transitions of living.

Look at the twists and turns in your life. Recognize how life's stages create new opportunities as well as new challenges.

Celebrate the changes of the seasons with a party on the first day of summer (June 21) or a vernal equinox tea on March 21.

Wise Words

Embracing change creates ease and freedom in your world.

The only constant is change.

Give yourself room for expansion. Give yourself room to change.

Allow change to happen to you. Don't resist it.

Sunrise and sunset are obvious reminders of change.

May we learn to accept life's constant changes.

The Only Constant Is Change

Intention

To illustrate the fact that nothing lasts forever.

Approximate Length

3 minutes

Lesson

The present situation can change in an instant. The yogi stays tranquil and accepts life's frequent turn of events while knowing that pleasure, pain, good, and bad never last forever.

Here's a parable that shows how quickly life can turn around.

There once was a farmer who had a magnificent prize-winning stallion. The farmer planned to sell him to a wealthy businessman for a large profit. One week before the horse was to be sold, a hurricane swept through the farmer's land. It tore down the barn where the horse was kept, and the stallion ran off. "What bad luck!" the farmer's wife said.

"Good luck, bad luck, who knows? We'll have to see," said the farmer.

The next week, the farmer and his wife saw a herd of horses galloping toward the farm. It was their stallion, leading four horses behind him. "What good luck!" said the farmer's wife.

"Good luck, bad luck, who knows? We'll have to see," said the farmer.

Soon the farmer and his son were training the new horses. One day the son was thrown by one of the horses and broke both his legs. The farmer's wife was very upset. "My only son! We never should have let those horses in. This is very bad luck," she said.

"Good luck, bad luck, who knows? We'll have to see," said the farmer.

The next week, soldiers came to the farm. Their king had declared war, and the soldiers were drafting every young man in the country. After seeing that the farmer's son had two broken legs, the soldiers left him at home. The farmer's wife was relieved. "Oh, what good luck we have!" she said.

As expected, the farmer said, "Good luck, bad luck, let's wait and see . . ."

The story illustrates how the farmer was a yogi in his understanding of change, staying detached from life's ups and downs. Change is the only thing we can be sure of, so why not accept it?

Let's accept and be thankful for what is true in our bodies and in our minds at this moment on this day. Know that change can be just a breath away.

Asanas for Deepening

Deliberately take your time with these postures, and notice change in all levels of your being. The posture may become much more comfortable for a while (good luck?) then change again (bad luck?)! Notice how the energy of the body continues to change with every breath.

At the start of asana practice, do the reclining hamstring stretch using a strap under the ball of the extended leg or, for the more flexible, the big-toe hold. Do it again at the end of class to feel the difference in the character of your muscles and your energy.

Sit in the over-and-under pose and invite your hips to melt into the earth. Take in the changing sensation. Can you sense softening or resistance?

Navasana (seated boat) will challenge your balance, the temperament of your hamstrings, and your breath.

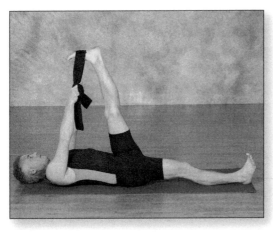
Reclining hamstring stretch

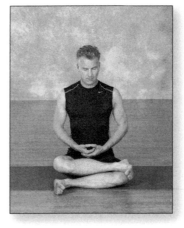
Over-and-under pose

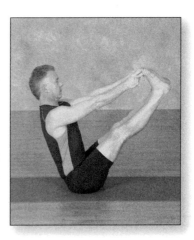
Navasana

Practice Off the Mat

Think of the impermanence in your life. The groceries you bought a few days ago, the children you raised, even the headache you had this morning, are now gone. Impermanence simply means that *everything* changes. The sages believe that if we are aware of the constant fluctuations of life, we'll be open, available, and ready for anything.

Consider the times in your life when bad luck has really been good luck in disguise. Judy shared this story about her coworker friend who left her job to work for another company. Judy missed her and believed that she couldn't do her job without her. A month later, Judy discovered that not only was her friend's replacement an excellent coworker but she also became her friend. Judy now has two friends where there was only one.

The waiting room at the doctor's office is filled. Is this good luck or bad luck? An extra 10 minutes gives you time to take in a pranayama practice to clear your mind and lower your blood pressure right before it's taken!

Wise Words

Change is the great educator of the cosmos.

It is only through changing circumstances that we learn and grow.

Life is a neverending spiral of change.

Don't attach to an outcome, because the outcome *will* change.

Surprise is a state of mind.

Fear

Intention

To use the tools of yoga to deal with fear.

Approximate Length

3 minutes

Lesson

How do we as yogis deal with our internalized view of fear?

When fear takes over our lives, we are less willing to take risks. This shuts down the third chakra, the solar plexus, the center of our will, power, and inner strength. When this chakra becomes deficient, we tend to close ourselves off to life's unlimited potential. Living a fearful existence will most assuredly keep your spirit at bay.

As yogis, we take a pragmatic view of the world, understanding that fear and uncertainty are parts of human existence. Whether you lived in a cave thousands of years ago fearing the attack of a lion, or whether you live in New York fearing another September 11, violence and suffering have always been part of this world.

So what kind of practice should we have if we live in fear of bombings, muggings, or even the more mundane events of life such as job interviews or confrontations with store clerks? Is there a breathing exercise that can help us through a panic attack? Are there tools for this?

The yoga path itself is the tool for the liberation of suffering. The practices of asana and pranayama are two of the most powerful tools for releasing the fear, anxiety, and anger that get locked in the body's tissues.

Our practices today will allow us to reconnect and balance our solar plexus and open the armor that covers the heart center chakra. When these chakras are open, we can connect with the priorities of the present moment, with gratitude and love. Then, instead of letting fear lead you, closing you off from life as it keeps you in a self-imposed prison, you can fill your heart with life force and live to the fullest extent.

Asanas for Deepening

Depending on levels of fear, it may be best to begin with a series of gentle backbends, untying the armor around the solar plexus and heart. Backbends stimulate circulation in the spine and make us feel more vital and alive. Almost any backbend can be tamed to nurture this effort: unsupported bhujangasana (cobra, no arms, photo *a*), setu bandha sarvangasana (bridge, photo *b*), shalabhasana (half locust, photo *c*), lunge (photo *d*), or standing backbend with hands supporting the lower waist (photo *e*).

Practice ustrasana (camel), focusing on opening the solar plexus and heart center. In the final stages, imagine your heart lifting out of its cage and flourishing with love, compassion, and inner wisdom. Let prana circulate and bring energy to those areas. Camel also helps relieve depression caused by anxiety.

Crow balances the third chakra and develops courage. Have fun and don't bother with whether you can complete the final pose; try lifting one foot at a time until you can maintain balance. If you are worried about falling on your face, put a pillow or blanket in front of you.

Gentle Backbends

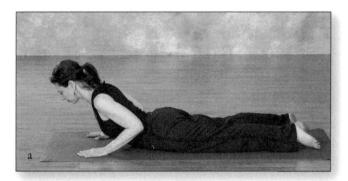

Bhujangasana

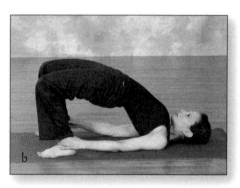

Setu bandha sarvangasana

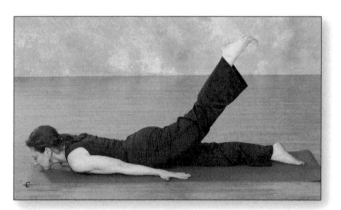

Shalabhasana

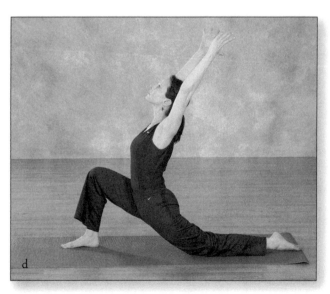

Lunge

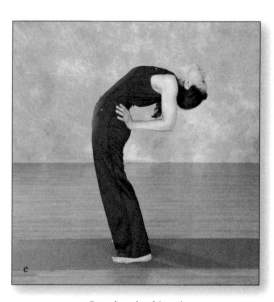

Standing backbend

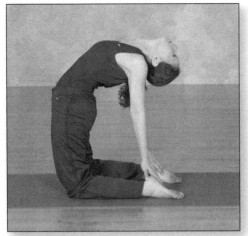

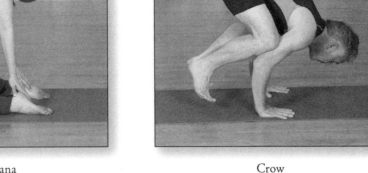

Ustrasana   Crow

Practice Off the Mat

The most important thing to do when you're in the midst of an anxiety attack or when you feel one coming on is to immediately stop what you're doing and catch your breath. At the moment of mindfulness of the anxiety attack, practice two-to-one breathing, in which the exhale is approximately twice as long as the inhale. Follow with four to eight rounds (six breaths per round) of nadi shodhana, breathing out of the left nostril.

When you feel frightened, imagine lying on the sand of a warm, tropical beach. With your exhalation, feel a wave pass down through the body, carrying away waste, fatigue, and worry. With the inhalation, a fresh wave passes up through the body, carrying energy and well-being from an ocean of cosmic vitality. Breathe this way 10 times.

Have you been closing off your spirit in an effort to protect it? Meditate on the heart center, where fear can get locked. Imagine that you are holding the key, and unlock the gate of the heart, feeling the fear and anxiety escape. By meditating on the heart center, we become attuned to deep-seated emotions and reconnect to life as it really is.

If fear of a situation is taking over your thoughts, think about the worst possible outcome. What happens? What bodily sensations arise? When you hit rock bottom, you can only go up. By thinking of the worst rather than denying or suppressing the result, we can move more easily through the fear that restricts our life force and keeps us locked in our self-induced prison.

Wise Words

We cannot change the world, only ourselves.

Through mindful practice, we develop concentration that leads to strength of mind.

Death comes to all of us. Knowing that death is part of life—just take a look at nature—will bring you a new appreciation of life. Recognition and gratitude for the now will naturally flourish.

Letting Go

Intention

To identify the importance of giving up emotional baggage.

Approximate Length

3 minutes

Lesson

How many of us are carrying emotional baggage from years ago? Here's a parable about carrying excess baggage.

Two monks were walking down a road toward a river with the intention of crossing it. The monks saw a woman at the riverbank who was waiting for someone to help her get across. This was centuries ago, and in those days, monks were forbidden to have any contact with women. The first monk said to the second monk, "That woman needs help. Shall we take her across the river with us?" The second monk angrily replied, "We can't do that. We'd be breaking our sacred vows!" The first monk thought about what his friend said, then took the woman on his back and carried her across the river. After traveling across and walking a long distance, the second monk, who was distraught about his brother monk's contact with the woman, went on and on about how the vows were now broken. What were they to do? How would they explain this back at the monastery? The first monk stopped, looked at the second monk, and said, "Brother, I left that woman two miles back. Why are you still carrying her?"

The yama aparigraha, nonpossessiveness, can teach us a lot about letting go of baggage. When we hold on to our outdated ideas, our way of doing things, and our negative circumstances, we hold on to things that we no longer need to carry.

The next time you feel yourself attached to an idea of how things should be, notice what effect the attachment has in your body. Do your muscles tighten? Does the breath feel stifled? Is your face tense?

Today our intention is the practice of letting go. Think of your yoga mat as a sacred place where you can unearth your buried baggage and give it to the universe. Only by letting go, forgiving, and letting guilt and anger fade away can we live in the moment and let the possibilities of life lead us.

Asanas for Deepening

In kurmasana (tortoise), surrender to the outcome. Let the stretch, breath, and open state of mind lead you. Be patient and notice how the mind begins to let go of its clutches.

Sit in baddha konasana (bound angle) with a brick between your feet, and choose the perfect moment to let go. Don't be in a rush to come out of the pose.

During the reclining twist, practice the willingness to be present and to let things happen.

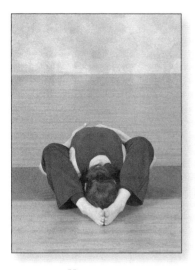
Kurmasana

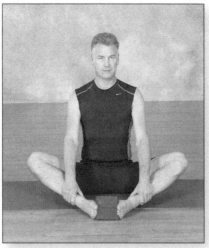
Baddha konasana

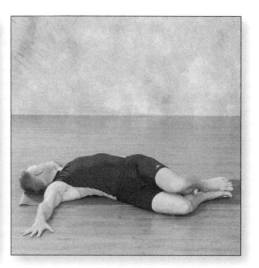
Reclining twist

Practice Off the Mat

Do you always have to get the last word in? Try letting someone else do it.

If you have children, pick your battles. Choose the battles that are most important; let go of everything else. Childhood, like all of life, is a stage.

If you always want to drive so that you can be in control, your practice is to let someone else do it.

Are you still carrying a grudge over a disagreement with a friend, relative, or business associate? Is there someone you haven't spoken to in years? Do you feel the same guilt, heartbreak, or anger as you did when it happened? Is there any reason why you still need to carry this burden? Let it go once and for all. This doesn't necessarily mean that you're letting this person back in your life. It simply means that you're able to move on.

Wise Words

Surrender is believing that we have done all that we can. It is trusting that things will work out.

Letting go means accepting your life without resistance.

When we practice releasing the past, we discover the authentic self within us.

Stay centered. Centering teaches us how to be compassionate with ourselves and flexible with our thoughts.

Patience

Intention

To recognize impatience in our lives and in our yoga practice.

Approximate Length

4 minutes

Lesson

It seems that of all the negative emotions we deal with, impatience is the most prominent. We see it in toddlers, business people, parents, seniors, everyone. You probably even see it in your yoga practice.

Impatience manifests itself in all kinds of ways. A friend of mine was waiting at a popular pizza place to pick up her order. It was a busy Sunday evening with wall-to-wall people waiting to pick up their pizzas. She noticed how demanding and impatient the man next to her was. He kept whispering under his breath, "Where's my damn pizza?" Finally, when his name was called, he yelled at the counterman, "This is a disgrace!" He shouted loudly enough so that all the customers could hear him say, "You said it would be ready by six o'clock!" The counterman apologetically said, "I'm sorry you've been waiting so long, sir, but it *is* six o'clock." "No, it's not!" the man shouted back. "It's 6:05!"

My pizza-less friend laughed at the absurdity of this scenario. Yet, how many of us can honestly say we've *never* been this steamed with impatience?

As a society, we suffer with impatience because our actions are uncontrolled and out of tune with the reality of the now. Our minds are preoccupied with the worries and anxieties of yesterday or tomorrow, and it's difficult to involve ourselves in the present. Rather than live in the moment, we find ourselves wanting things to be faster, better, and smoother. It's as though we're in a cosmic disagreement with the way things are actually happening.

Our yoga practice provides one of the best and most systematic approaches to regaining our patience. Asanas bring us back in touch with the physical body. We begin to feel again. We begin to notice those bodily sensations of impatience. We learn how to wait and how to let our bodies open at their own pace.

During today's practice, when impatience-driven anxiety comes up, rather than push the thoughts away, be mindful that they are part of the moment. Like all moments, this one will pass.

Patience is a form of wisdom. It helps us accept that everything evolves in its own time.

Asanas for Deepening

Over time, the body unfolds. If you honor exploration and patience, you discover how everything changes all the time. This is the basis of learning to live in the moment.

Don't rush past the early stages of paschimottanasana (seated forward bend), waiting to get somewhere you're not naturally ready to be. Find your first place of resistance and adapt before going any further. Once you're settled, bring your attention to where you feel the breath in your body. From that place, follow the movement of each inhalation and exhalation. Notice what comes up. Are you calm? Does the mind wander? Is this a place of clarity for you? When feelings of impatience come up, bring yourself back to the movement of the breath.

During vasisthasana (side plank), take the posture in as many stages as necessary. Try it first with the bottom knee on the floor (photo *a*). Then extend the legs (photo *b*), first practicing balance. Finally, extend the top arm strongly upward (photo *c*).

In balasana (child's pose), take a deep, full breath into the muscles of your back and hum your exhalation. The vibration and sound through the body is powerful medicine.

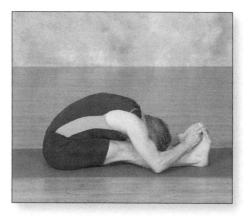

Paschimottanasana

Vasisthasana

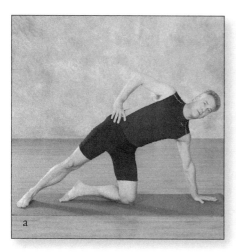

One knee on ground

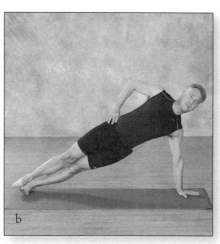

Legs extended

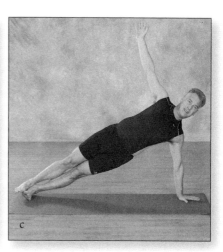

Legs and top arm extended

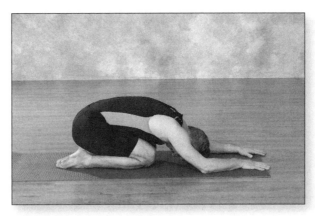
Balasana

Practice Off the Mat

Next time you are in a restaurant waiting for an order, think about the man and his pizza. Then ask yourself, can I wait five minutes for *my* pizza?

Sometimes the best practice is to watch what others do. The man at the pizza place was able to awaken my friend to the impatience in the world. If you have a friend, relative, or coworker who acts with impatience, spend some time with this person with the intention of looking at his or her impatient characteristics. Without judging or trying to change this person, find out what makes this person impatient. Look at his or her physical reactions, and listen to his or her tone of voice. Learning to identify another person's negative emotions will help you recognize them in yourself. If you maintain your sense of the moment with clarity and calm, you'll be setting an excellent example.

The world is full of places to practice patience: in traffic jams, in the long line at the bank, store, or pizza place, or in the office waiting for someone to e-mail a reply or return your call.

Do you interrupt others when they're speaking? Do you find your mind moving faster than the speed of light, your words unable to wait? Next time this happens, first become aware of it, then try to pause and really listen to the other person speaking. You may find that you're missing half the conversation!

When you feel impatient, try a quick, calm breath. Exhale to a mental count of seven and hold for four. Inhale to a mental count of four and hold for four. Practice four cycles. Adjust your count if the breath length feels shallow.

Wise Words

It's said that much of our discontent with life comes from not fully experiencing life exactly as it happens.

Impatience is a defensive response to a situation that isn't going our way.

When we experience the calmness that results from our yoga practices, we become more centered, satisfied, and patient.

Our thoughts can overwhelm our perception of the present moment because the mind is too busy focusing on the future or on the past. Impatience arises because events are not moving as fast as our thoughts.

We need to realize that in order to expand our level of patience, we must learn to accommodate the moment.

Chapter 10
Mindfulness

Do not dwell in the past; do not dream of the future.
Concentrate the mind on the present moment.

—Buddha

Have you ever driven somewhere and missed the scenery completely? You did the driving but didn't bother to look around.

Think of other experiences you've missed because you didn't pay attention. When we apply mindfulness to daily activities such as driving, brushing our teeth, or eating our morning bowl of cereal, our life becomes a moving meditation.

The lessons that follow will illustrate moving into mindfulness by paying attention. Once mindfulness is at the top of your mind, you'll be amazed at how much of life you have missed. As the saying goes, "Those who are awake live in a state of amazement."

Mindfulness: The Core of Practice

Intention

To integrate mindfulness into practice.

Approximate Length

2 minutes

Lesson

It's said by many that in order to practice yoga, you don't have to be flexible or strong, you just have to be awake. Mindfulness is the core of yoga practice. It is what separates practicing asana from just another stretch. Mindfulness means fully experiencing what happens in the here and now. It's the art of becoming deeply aware of the present moment.

Mindfulness means doing one thing at a time. We put our full attention into what we're doing—whether it is our yoga practice, driving the car, or talking to our friends—so that we can be awake in that moment.

When we're mindful, we're not missing what's happening now by thinking about the past or future. Our inner focus is in charge; distractions stay on the periphery of the mind. Focus stays intact, and our immediate experience is fully realized.

The emotional benefits of mindfulness are boundless. It helps us turn down the noise in our heads—feelings of anger or doubt, worries about tomorrow, clinging to the past.

In our practice, mindfulness begins by feeling the pose come to life, sensing the response of the breath, being mindful of stretch, strength, and balance as well as of our boundaries.

Lie in shavasana. Pay attention to your breath. Let your mind become absorbed in the sound of the inhale and the sound of the exhale. As if you're watching the waves of the ocean, let your mind be drawn into the presence and stillness. The breathing is always changing. No single breath is the same as the last.

Asanas for Deepening

Practice postures using an internal mantra. This could be any set of words that has meaning to you. If you don't have a mantra, use an affirmation such as "I am strong" or "Practice patience." The mantra can be inhaled and exhaled, such as "Let" on the inhale, "go" on the exhale.

Begin with surya namaskara (sun salutation) (see pages 58-59). When flowing through postures, be mindful of the muscular action, like a full-body stocking. Hug your muscles to the bones, and draw your energy toward the midline of the body. Try not to miss anything here, not a joint, a muscle, or a thought.

In natarajasana (king dancer), breathe smoothly, and bring the pose to life. Support your mindfulness with prana. Accept where you are in this moment without striving, without comparing, and without judging.

Finish with reclining leg cradles. When you can't pull the leg in any tighter, stay where you are. Maintain the action of the pose and relax with the intensity of the stretch. Close your eyes and let go into who you really are.

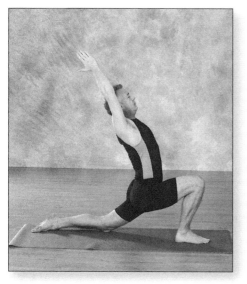

Surya namaskara

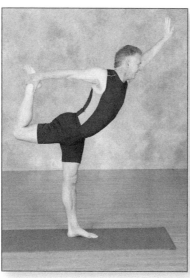

Natarajasana

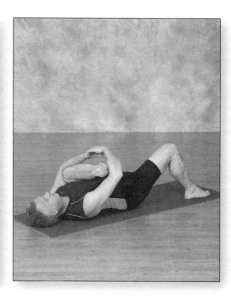

Reclining leg cradles

Practice Off the Mat

Allow mindfulness to seep into your actions when you brush your teeth, wash the dishes, talk on the phone, or taste that first sip of morning tea.

One-step meditation. Whenever you feel yourself becoming unfocused or too busy to concentrate, try the one-step meditation. This is a walking meditation that's done while walking very slowly, one step at a time. Each time you take a forward step, mentally say, *One*. As the opposite foot comes forward, mentally say, *Step*. As you do this, take in all that's happening at that moment—how the feet feel as they touch the ground, how the knee joints feel when they bend, how the weight shifts from left to right. Mindfulness, like all things of merit, can be accomplished one step at a time.

Mindfulness of breath. Count each set of in-and-out breaths as one until you reach 10. The object is not to get to 10 but to become aware of how much the mind rambles into the past and future. Bring yourself back to the present, the only place where there is truly any control.

Wise Words

Practice mindfulness during your daily living to encourage you to stop and smell the roses.

Yoga is the method by which the restless mind is calmed and its energy is directed into constructive channels.

Be mindful because this moment will pass. If you are somewhere else, you will not have lived it.

Paying Attention

Intention

To learn objectivity of the mind; to take a step toward meditation.

Approximate Length

2 minutes

Lesson

According to yoga philosophy, the world is exactly as it needs to be. This means that everything that happens to us personally and globally, whether we like it or not, is exactly what is supposed to be happening. Our mindfulness practice, regardless of whether we're planting tulips or practicing triangle, is about noticing when we're not paying attention.

When you begin to notice and pay attention to life as it is, spiritual questions begin to arise. In the yogic tradition, they can only be worked out through clear thinking.

Our asana practice imparts the importance of the present, to be in the moment whether we are depressed or anxious or calm or tired. This gives us the means to become aware of vrittis, the fluctuations of the mind. We begin by learning first to focus on the gross aspects of the body and then on the more discriminating components of prana, as well as on our ability to control it.

Gradually we begin to develop the mind's capacity to focus on one thing—this is called dharana, the concentration one needs in order to meditate and the sixth limb of Raja yoga. From here, the mind instinctively flows into dhyana, meditation, the seventh limb of Raja yoga.

Today our intention is the eternal practice of training the mind to pay attention, that is, to wake up to life both internally and externally.

Asanas for Deepening

In all postures, work with the internal mantra "breathing, grounding, lengthening." Exhale, breathing down to the toes. Inhale up to the crown of the head, feeling and sensing the breath move through you.

During inverted table, feel the hands and feet strongly reaching down, spine lengthening in both directions, shoulders opening and moving away from each other.

In matsyasana (fish), the chest continues to lift through the pose. The lungs are engaged in the awareness of breath, and the spine lifts into the back.

In padmasana (lotus or half lotus), the weight of the body sinks into the earth. Awaken the crown of the head and allow it to rise to the heavens. Expand the body; expand the mind. Step away from the thinking process and simply watch what unfolds.

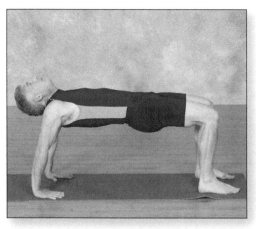

Inverted table

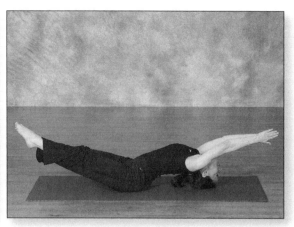

Matsyasana

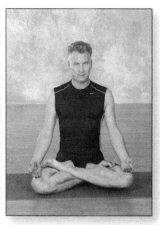

Padmasana

Practice Off the Mat

[This practice can be done anywhere at anytime and is a highly recommended technique for aspiring meditators.] Sit with your eyes closed. Just sit. Focus your attention on your breath, on a mantra, or on a focus point such as a candle or a deity.

What happens? Do you notice a pain in your back? Do you hear your breath? Do you feel your heart beating? Are you thirsty? Just feel that. Where does the mind go? Are you frustrated, impatient, tired, calm? Try to just witness these thoughts and sensations without changing or judging them.

See how long you can sit in mindfulness. Now open your eyes and reveal what has just happened. How long were you able to sit before your thoughts clouded the open spaces of your mind? The more you practice, the more quickly you can step back from your thoughts and simply be the observer.

Wise Words

In yoga asana, we live from moment to moment in the sensation; we are one with the feeling.

What do we do with our available prana? We can devour loads of mental energy by unknowingly allowing thoughts to drift to other places and people.

It's through continuous and vigilant practice that we develop the objectivity of the mind.

Dharana

Intention

To learn concentration.

Approximate Length

1 minute

Lesson

Dharana is the sixth limb of Raja yoga. The objective of this limb is to hold our concentration in one direction. When we apply dharana, we highlight a particular activity of the mind. The brighter it becomes, the more the other activities of the mind fall away. This practice stops the mind from rambling by willfully holding it on a focus point such as a mantra, the breath, or a point on the body.

The attention to internal-body adjustments during each pose brings one-pointed awareness to the muscles, joints, and organs. But they also turn the mind's focus to the present moment. When we consciously drop the shoulders, the mind becomes present. When the mind wanders, the shoulders rise. These adjustments tell the mind, "Be here, not somewhere else."

The technique of dharana in asana helps us learn to integrate the control of the breath and prana within the body. The practice naturally leads to concentration and to strength in our emotional body.

Asanas for Deepening

During virabhadrasana II (warrior II), bring your drishti (focus point) to the tip of the second finger of the hand you are facing, keeping it steady, as if the awareness of the pose depends on it.

To get into candle, squat on the toes with your hands in prayer position over the head. Release any exertion or tension, and let the legs support you. Flow with whatever may happen, and focus the mind on the toes.

In upavistha konasana (seated angle), free yourself of any uneasiness along the length of your spine. Feel for more subtle areas of tension, and use your breath to soften and relax while moving toward deep concentration.

Reclining (photo *a*) and seated (photo *b*) virasana (hero) are poses of stillness, and they cultivate inner stability. Many use seated hero as a meditation posture. Apply the breath to gently express the meaning of the posture. Exhale and feel the pelvic bones drop into the earth. Inhale and draw up the front of the spine, lifting the soft tissues at the front of your spine.

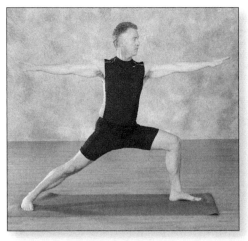

Virabhadrasana II

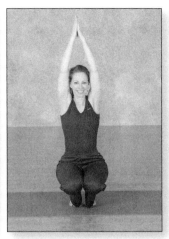

Candle

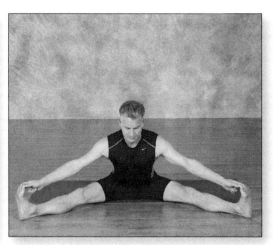

Upavistha konasana

Virasana

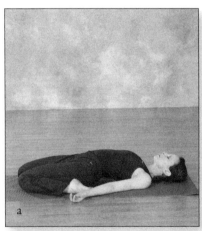

a

Reclining

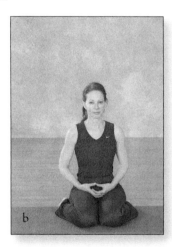

b

Seated

Practice Off the Mat

Yoga philosophy teaches us that if we want to live a contented existence, we have to break the patterns that keep us running from discomfort or unpleasantness.

To practice dharana, or concentration, become aware of the breath. Place your attention on your abdomen, then let it rest lightly inside on top of the diaphragm muscle. Once you can feel the breath, don't concern yourself with the way you breathe. Instead, simply let the breath move through you as you watch it.

Try not to miss a breath: breathing out, breathing in. If the mind wanders off the path, don't get stuck on a thought. Instead, gently bring your mind back and begin again. Your only objective is to surrender to the movement of the breath. Let it come; let it go. Each inhale, each exhale, move it on through.

If you thread this practice into your day—at work, while working at your computer, while sitting in a waiting room, virtually anywhere—you will begin to experience the benefits of santosha, or contentment.

Wise Words

Dharana, or concentration, is preparation for dhyana, or meditation.

When the mind has become purified by yoga practices, we experience inner healing.

The moment we start to force, we begin to lose awareness of the nervous system or the situation.

When you lose your concentration, each time bring the attention back to the object of focus.

During asana, ask yourself, "Where am I? Where is my focus? Can I take it deeper?"

When we begin to truly listen to our minds, we experience the waterfall of distractions. Simply observe and watch one thought fall into another.

Mindfulness of Gratitude

Intention

To live in a state of gratitude.

Approximate Length

5 to 7 minutes

Lesson

Mindfulness of gratitude is a powerful practice. Practicing mindfulness of gratitude guides us to an immediate realization that our lives are developing within a larger context.

A gratitude practice is particularly beneficial to those who are troubled with mild depression or who are carrying feelings of negativity about situations in their lives. Some choose a melancholy existence because they don't know any other way.

Our asana practice helps us appreciate the miracle of the body. Remember, it's important to be grateful for having two legs and two arms—and a brain to boot!

When we make asana a daily practice, a natural antidepressant kicks in. With mindful breathing, our anxiety levels decrease, endorphins are released, and our mood lifts. The more we practice, the deeper we relax.

Quieting the mind and generating a strong connection with the heart add regenerative energy and an attitude of gratitude to your entire system.

Today we begin our practice with the Gratitude of Heart breath. This is like an adjustment for our feelings; when we focus on gratitude, appreciation, compassion, or another positive, loving emotion, our heart rhythms immediately shift. Blood pressure normalizes. Stress hormones drop. The immune system gets stronger. During difficult times, Gratitude of Heart breath can help ease depression and anxiety.

The essential step in the Gratitude of Heart breath is to energetically send out appreciation or love. Feeling these emotions creates a cascade of biochemical events that nourish the body and mind. Emotionally we feel calm, clear, and strong.

This is an exceptional way to begin our asana practice because so much of what we do in our poses requires awareness and an opening of the heart center.

First close your eyes and let the body relax. Shift from the outside world to the inside world, and gently bring your attention to the area around your heart, the mid-chest. Put your right hand on your heart. Envision your breath going in and out through the heart center. Take very slow, intentional deep breaths.

Now visualize something that's effortless for you to appreciate: your children, friends, parents, God, pets. Send them genuine gratitude and love as you breathe through your heart. Really feel the emotion, not just the thought.

After you've finished the heart breath, try to hold on to those qualities of appreciation and love as long as you can. This acts as a buffer against recurring stress or anxiety.

Asanas for Deepening

Bound baddha konasana (bound butterfly) opens the chest, quiets the mind, and helps relieve anxiety and stress.

During seated yoga mudra, succumb to an attitude of admiration for life as you practice.

In bhujangasana (cobra), feel the spine opening, the collarbone lengthening outward, and the chest opening in the heart center. Notice the prana concentrated in the front and back of the heart. Breathe with compassion and gratitude.

Chakrasana (wheel) improves circulation, stimulates the nervous system, and generates a feeling of well-being. It also increases energy and counteracts depression.

If tripod comes naturally to you, try tripod with the knee inside the opposite knee. Put one knee into the back of the other knee. Then make sure you pause to marvel at the wonder of your amazing body! Follow with child's pose.

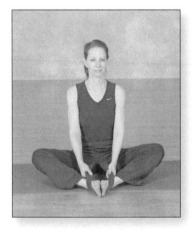

Bound baddha konasana

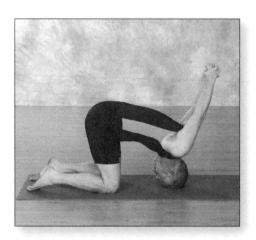

Seated yoga mudra

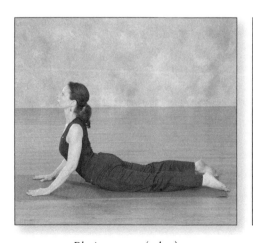

Bhujangasana (cobra)

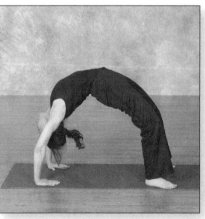

Chakrasana

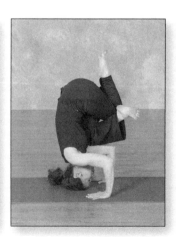

Tripod variation

Practice Off the Mat

Keep a gratitude journal. Every evening at bedtime, write down five things you are grateful for. You may want to go with the obvious—your health, family, or job—but the entries can be as simple (although just as important) as having running water, clean clothes, or the beauty of a rosebud. Within a week, you'll find that your daily gratitude level will heighten, your role in life will be more realistic, and your anxiety level will decrease. Perspective is powerful medicine!

For an entire day, be the messenger of good news. Every time you speak to someone, let it be of something pleasant or uplifting, and make a conscious effort to notice and acknowledge what's good about the day.

Wise Words

Every day is a gift. That's why it's called the present.

Living in appreciation makes every day better, and there is always something to appreciate.

May you be awake to the gifts you receive and give.

Holiday Gratitude

Intention

To feel gratitude in the heart.

Approximate Length

4 minutes

Lesson

[Recommended for use during Thanksgiving or holiday classes.] At this time of year, we're taught to count our blessings and to be grateful for what we have. But gratitude, like everything else, is a *choice*. When we choose to be grateful, we focus on the things that are right in our life as opposed to the things that are not, like what we can and cannot do physically in our asana practice. Applying this definition to gratitude, we begin to see our entire existence as a miracle rather than as just the passing of time.

The practice of gratitude is empowering. It can change the way you perceive your life.

Let's close our eyes, bring the hands in anjali mudra (namaste), and gently give our attention to the center of our chest, the heart center. Focus on the rising and falling of the chest as you breathe in and out. Think about the things in your life that fill you with happiness and joy—your friends, family, pets, or whatever you feel grateful for. As you focus on these things, you may begin to feel warm, calm, and content.

You are now in a state of gratitude.

Today, let's combine the powerful healing energies of asana with the practice of kindness, compassion, and gratitude. If you wish, send these healing energies to someone who needs them today.

Asanas for Deepening

Be grateful that you're able to come to yoga class to move and appreciate the miracle that we refer to as "the body." With this attitude of gratitude, any posture can be practiced with compassion and gratefulness.

Traditionally, balasana (child's pose) has been called "the pose of gratitude." This calming, steadying pose brings us into submission to the present, grounding us in ease and gratitude.

Kapotasana (resting pigeon) indulges the internal organs with natural massage. Be grateful for the strength of the diaphragm muscle that helps you breathe. With the forehead on the ground, the senses are less active, and the mind quickly becomes calm, the back of the heart soft. For a more profound effect, have a partner gently press on your lower back in order to help ease the hold you may have on your hips and sacrum.

For the horse pose, while on the knees, bring one heel to the oppostite hip and put your arms in garudasana (eagle). Both satisfying and humbling, horse pose is a colorful path to feeling the bountiful inner structure of the skeletal system.

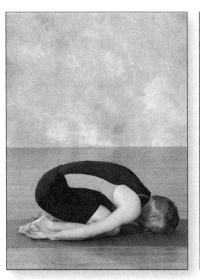

Balasana

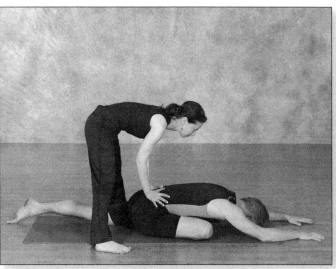

Kapotasana

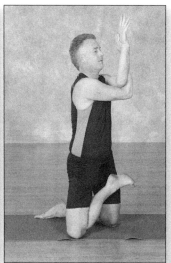

Horse pose

Practice Off the Mat

On a daily basis—not just during holidays—strengthen your spirit by being mindful of the blessings of your daily life.

At family gatherings such as holiday dinners, find a poem, prayer, or affirmation that speaks to you. Stand up at the dinner table and share it with your loved ones. While many families gather just to eat, you will have changed the shape of the holiday by planting the seeds of love, spirit, and gratitude.

Remind your children—and yourself—to be grateful for food, clothing, shelter, and love.

Never take anything or anyone for granted. As we learn from "The only constant is change" lesson, things that we have today may not be here tomorrow.

After spending time with a good friend, send him a card or an e-mail to let him know how special he is in your life.

Don't forget birthdays. Everyone gets one day a year to celebrate the day they came into this world. Celebrate yours with joy and enthusiasm.

Wise Words

Use your practice to look inward and experience what you are truly thankful and grateful for.

Notice how your yoga practice creates the spiritual qualities and well-being that puts us in touch with our dharma (life purpose).

A quiet mind gains access to inner wisdom. Listen to that wisdom and you'll know what feels most useful, fulfilling, and complete in your life.

Celebrate the ordinary.

Mindful Eating

Intention

To discover awareness and gratitude in eating.

Approximate Length

2 to 3 minutes

Lesson

Do you ever eat but taste only the first bite? You sit down at the table and put food into your mouth, but your mind is somewhere else. There's no connection between your mind and your mouth.

When we eat, we feed our inner selves. This requires a thoughtful approach because, after all, food sustains life. Eating calmly, with full awareness and gratitude, feeds the mind and spirit as well as the body.

Most students of yoga find that as the body becomes healthier, we naturally become more sensitive to *what* we eat and *how* we eat. This new awareness helps us make wise choices. From the yogic point of view, food has properties that influence our physical, mental, emotional, and spiritual life. Stale, processed, or overripe foods have lost their prana. Ingesting these foods leads to a state of dullness and lethargy. Foods with a lot of sugar or caffeine, such as chocolate and coffee, overstimulate the nervous and hormonal systems, and they counteract the balancing effects of our asana practice.

But foods that are as close to the earth as possible—fresh vegetables, whole grains, and fruits—are neither depressing nor stimulating. Like our asana and pranayama practice, they nourish and energize, bringing us into balance and harmony with our bodies, minds, and emotions.

It is also important to pay attention to how much we eat. Brahmacharya, moderation in all aspects of life, is encouraged in yoga. A yogi never comes to a point of complete satiation. Try to fill yourself to only three-fourths full at each meal, leaving room for healthy digestion.

When it comes to your relationship with food, the best advice is to enjoy it. If you devote yourself to the enjoyment and gratitude of the food itself and its source, you'll find out what truly nourishes you, and you'll no longer need what doesn't.

Asanas for Deepening

The asanas focus on postures that help food assimilate, digest, and eventually move through the system.

Supta sukhasana (reclining, easy, cross-legged pose) soothes heartburn (acid reflux) and improves digestion by increasing blood supply to the intestines.

Intestinal massage is excellent for improving elimination problems, including constipation. Sit on the heels. Start just above and inside the point of the pelvic bone at the right hip. Using the fists, massage gently up the right side of the abdomen where the ascending colon is. Continue across the diaphragm (upper abdominal area) to massage the transverse colon, and then move down the left side to complete the process on the descending colon. You should be able to feel (and possibly hear) gas bubbles and blockages being moved along. To enhance the pressure on the organs, bend forward while you continue to massage.

Matsyendrasana (half seated twist) massages and tones the internal organs and maintains space and mobility in the spine.

The change in gravity during sarvangasana (either the inverted action pose or the shoulderstand) affects the abdominal organs so that the bowels move freely.

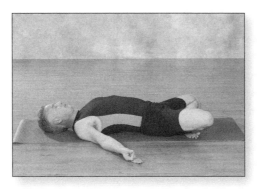

Supta sukhasana

Intestinal Massage

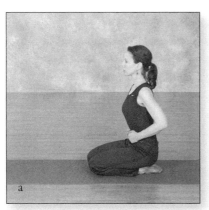

Fists at pelvic bones

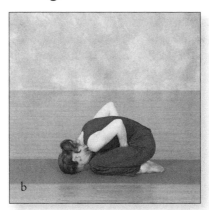

Forward bend

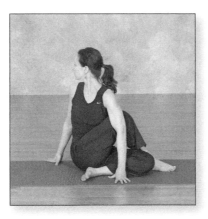

Matsyendrasana

Sarvangasana

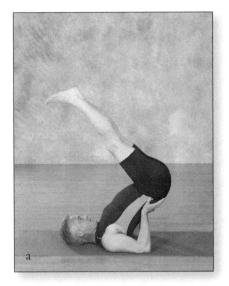

Inverted action pose

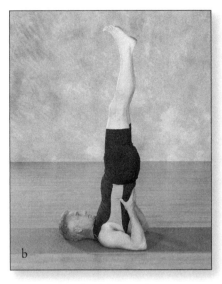

Shoulder stand

Practice Off the Mat

Follow a mindful eating practice. Start by eating a small piece of food, such as a raisin or a piece of popcorn, as slowly as possible. Savor the touch and taste of each morsel as you enjoy the sensation of food with total mindfulness.

Enjoy the flavors, colors, and textures of your meal. If we truly enjoy our food, we won't continue to eat mindlessly, in search of the enjoyment we aren't getting.

Eat alone and without any distractions such as the television or a newspaper. Simply sit, just you and your food, being attentive to the nourishment your body is receiving.

If you want to give your friends a meal they'll never forget, invite them over for a silent mindfulness dinner. Again make sure that there are no distractions such as music, television, or reading materials. This is especially interesting when you're eating crunchy foods, such as cereals or chips, or slurppy foods, such as stews and soups. Another twist on this technique is to eat in the dark!

Just for fun, try eating with the opposite hand or eating with chopsticks.

Wise Words

Take a moment before you eat to quietly give thanks, reflecting on the source of your food and its purpose in your life.

What is your food doing to you? Is it nourishing you? Is it stimulating you or is it making you sleepy? Can you judge when you're full, or do you overeat until you're stuffed?

Practicing mindfulness in asana teaches us to recognize the feeling of fullness.

Pay attention to what you are eating. Notice the effect of food in your life, and enjoy it as a gift.

Setting an Intention

Intention

To create a meaningful objective to hatha yoga practice.

Approximate Length

1 minute

Lesson

When we set our intentions for practice, we let self-observation be our first step. To set an intention requires an awareness of our current situation and ourselves. An intention can be simple, such as, "I need relief in the right side of my neck," or, "I've been working all day, and I want to clear my head." Or your intention may be more complex, such as, "I want to move out of a bad relationship, and I need the inner strength to do it," or, "I want to work on a challenging posture in order to develop my self-confidence."

Keep the intention concrete. Be specific. This will allow you to maintain focus in your practice. See yourself in complete mindfulness before taking the first conscious breath.

Asanas for Deepening

Spinal rocks (rocking chair) wake up the energy in the spine.

For arm stretch, sit in any seated posture. Stretch the arms out to the sides. Let the movement be carried by a deep inner energy rather than by just muscle power. Think of a loved one who you're trying to stretch out to. Notice how intention matters.

Relax into the full expression of inverted plank as you observe the responses and fluctuations among the outer body, will, and ego.

For hidden lotus, take padmasana (lotus) on the knees, then slowly walk your hands forward until the abdomen is on the ground.

For intention vinyasa, begin with balasana (child's pose, photo *a*). Move into adho mukha shvanasana (downward-facing dog, photo *b*) then urdhva mukha shvanasana (upward-facing dog, photo *c*). Finish with balasana (child's pose, photo *d*). Move with the breath. Think only of the synchronicity of the breath, not of the movement itself. If the breath is restricted in anyway, consciousness will also be restricted.

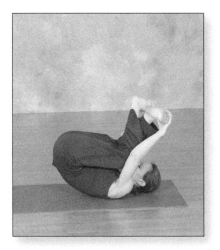

Spinal rocks

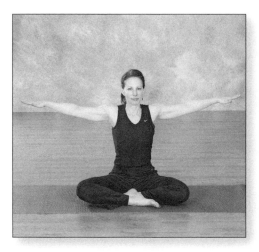

Arm stretch

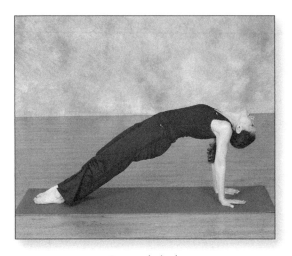

Inverted plank

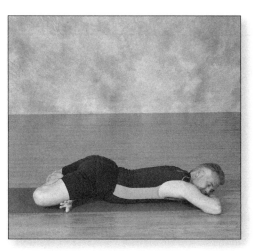

Hidden lotus

Intention Vinyasa

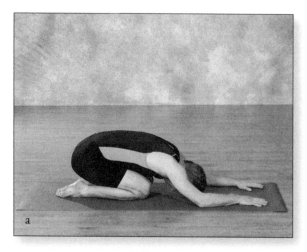

Balasana

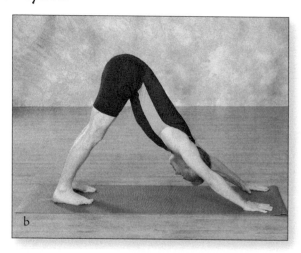

Adho mukha shvanasana

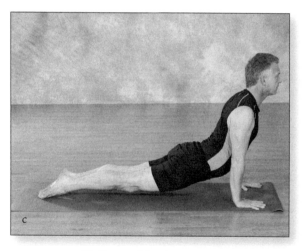

Urdhva mukha shvanasana

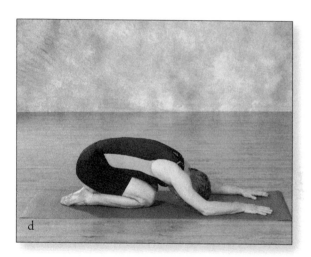

Balasana

Practice Off the Mat

During your day, set your intention for what you need to do. Bring your mind to the intention with full acceptance of the moment. Be sure to bring your breath, along with compassion for yourself, especially if it's something you don't enjoy doing, such as running errands. Before you begin, stop for a moment and breathe self-acceptance into your eyes, skin, muscles, bones, and heart. Breathe and receive.

Wise Words

Before you begin to move your body, pause to observe how you feel. Notice your physical sensations, the quality of your natural breath, and your state of mind.

You can practice the same pose every day for 10 years and, by applying mindful intention, have a different experience every time you do it.

Chapter 11
Chakras

Everything changes; nothing remains without change.

—Buddha

The chakras are the seven major energy centers that regulate the flow of subtle energy in our bodies. They're arranged vertically from the base of the spine to the top of the head.

Chakras

Chakra 1: Muladhara—Root

Chakra 2: Svadhisthana—Lower abdomen

Chakra 3: Manipura—Solar plexus

Chakra 4: Anahata—Heart center

Chakra 5: Visuddha—Throat center

Chakra 6: Ajna—Eyebrow center

Chakra 7: Sahasrara—Crown center

Chakra is the Sanskrit word for wheel. These "wheels" are spinning vortexes of energy.

As centers of life-force consciousness, chakras are the prominent areas through which we take in and disburse life energies. Through external and internal life situations, a chakra can either be lacking in energy or have too much of it, and therefore it can become imbalanced.

The lessons that follow introduce each chakra, its characteristics, its balances, and its imbalances. Learning about them gives us knowledge of our inner and outer worlds so that we can savor each chakra's positive experiences and reverse its negatives ones. The lessons are intended to awaken and balance these centers of consciousness in order to facilitate healing and to help us live a more fulfilling and meaningful life.

Chakra 1: Muladhara

Intention

To awaken and balance the root chakra.

Approximate Length

2 minutes

Lesson

The first chakra, the root chakra, is called muladhara. This is the building block on which all the other chakras rest. It's located at the perineum, midway between the anus and the genitals. It relates to the element of earth and vibrates to the color red.

The main consideration in the root chakra is survival. Only when our survival needs are met can we feel grounded and safe in our lives. If this chakra is imbalanced, any growth will be without roots, therefore lacking the stability necessary for long-term change.

When this chakra is balanced, we have good physical energy and health, as well as a sense of groundedness. We feel comfortable in our bodies, and we feel a sense of safety and security. When this chakra is extreme, we have an impression of heaviness, we're sluggish and slow to move. We tend to overeat. We also resist change. If this chakra is lacking energies, we feel spacey, insecure, fearful, and anxious, and we have a tendency to be underweight.

Our physical imbalances manifest as aches and pains in the legs, feet, and bones, and problems with the body's elimination system. A person with an excessive first chakra may experience constipation; a person whose first chakra is lacking energy may experience diarrhea.

Today our practice will focus on noticing gravity. We will move slowly and deeply in order to feel all aspects of the body and to sense the body's roots in the earth.

Asanas for Deepening

Begin with foot stomping. Stomp the feet in order to open the foot chakras.

Emphasize standing poses. Standing postures such as Utkatasana (chair) help open and strengthen the lower body and focus root attention downward.

Chant, "Lam," the seed sound of muladhara, with movement. Combine uttanasana (standing forward bend) with the seed sound *lam* as you exhale down to the earth. Bend the knees if your fingertips don't touch the ground. Repeat three to six times.

Perform asvini mudra. Begin with makarasana (crocodile) with your legs together. Exhale and contract the buttocks and pull in the anal sphincter muscles. Inhale and relax completely. This helps strengthen and energize the muscles around the base of the spine and pelvic floor and it brings awareness to the root.

Finish with mula bandha (root lock), a prolonged contraction of the muscles at the perineum. The contraction changes the flow of prana (subtle energy) in the body by reversing the downward moving energy in the root chakra, causing it to move upward. Holding energy here is stabilizing and calming, and it enhances concentration.

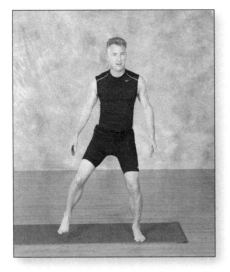

Foot stomping

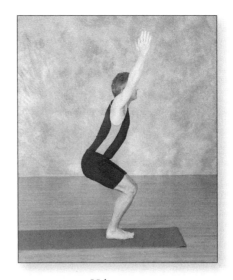

Utkatasana

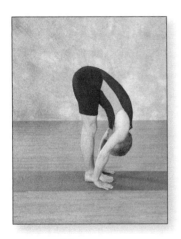

Uttanasana

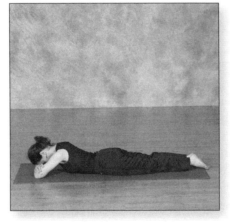

Asvini mudra

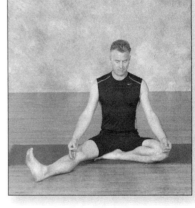

Mula bandha

Practice Off the Mat

To increase first-chakra energy, eat proteins and earthy foods such as root vegetables. Spend time outdoors. Ride a bike, power walk, or garden. Tune in to your body.

To decrease root-chakra energy, lighten up and smile. Eat organic, fresh, and live foods as opposed to processed food. Sleep less, and increase the movements of the body.

Wise Words

Muladhara means support or foundation.

Our experiences in the world can only be accomplished when we are able to meet our most basic survival issues of safety and security.

When muladhara chakra is healthy and balanced, we feel nurtured and experience our connection to the whole.

Chakra 2: Svadhisthana

Intention

To awaken and work through imbalances in the second chakra.

Approximate Length

4 minutes

Lesson

Svadhisthana, the second chakra, is located at the lower abdomen and corresponds to the sacral vertebrae. This area links into the sciatic nerve and is the center of motion for the body. Svadhisthana relates to the element of water and vibrates to the color orange.

Our motivating principle in chakra two is pleasure. Once survival needs are met in chakra one, we turn toward enjoyment. When this chakra is balanced, we experience happiness, joy, and sensuality; we have a passion for life; we're expressive, trusting, and sexually satisfied.

Imbalance of this chakra causes feelings of guilt, powerlessness, insecurity, isolation, and oversensitivity. There's usually a blaming of the self and of others, emotional instability, and manipulative behavior. When this chakra is overactive, we may have sexual addictions or obsessive attachments, crave stimulation, and be excessively sensitive. When this chakra is lacking, we may feel fearful of change, have poor social skills, be stiff in the body and in life, or have guilty feelings.

Physical symptoms of imbalance manifest in the sex organs, large intestines, pelvis, hips, and bladder. Some common physical manifestations of imbalance are impotence, frigidity, infertility, and lower back pain.

Today our practice for opening and balancing the second chakra involves working with movement in the hips and lower abdomen. When practicing, keep in mind the balanced second chakra; experiencing the joy and pleasure in the body and in life. Move fluidly, like water, being sensitive to sensation.

Asanas for Deepening

Begin with standing pelvic tilts. Connect with earth energy through the legs and move it into the second chakra. Tilt the pelvis forward as you push against the earth. Imagine that the energy you're building in the legs is flowing like water into your sacral area.

Combine baddha konasana (butterfly) forward bends with a chant. As you bend forward in bandha konasana, chant the second chakra seed sound *vam* as you exhale and hold the posture. Repeat three to six times. As you bend forward, bring awareness to the pleasure center.

Move into pelvic rotations with bhastrika breath (bellows breath). From a seated position, make clockwise pelvic rotations and begin the bhastrika breath. Visualize stirring up the life force in the second chakra. Be sure to rotate in the opposite direction.

Finish in reclining virasana (hero). Lift the arms overhead, relax, and tune into a vibrant orange pulsation within the lower abdomen. Allow the abdomen to gently open.

Standing Pelvic Tilts

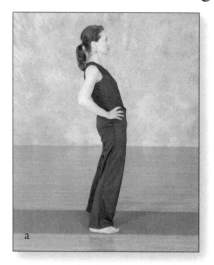

Tilt pelvis forward

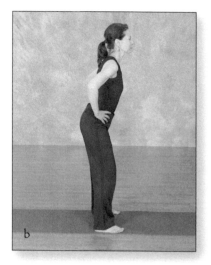

Tilt pelvis back

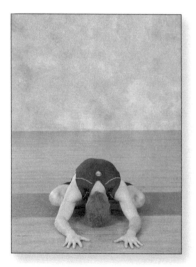

Baddha konasana

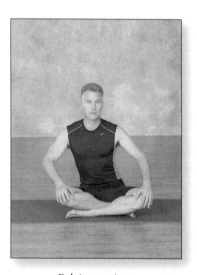

Pelvic rotations

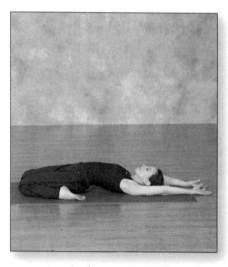

Reclining virasana

Practice Off the Mat

Drink water. To unleash stuck energy, we have to be able to move and change. This is the principal purpose of the second chakra, to move energy along.

Move. Walk, dance, run, stretch. Go with the flow of your body.

Rediscover your sexuality. Fill your sexual journey with passion and romance. Allow it to be more than just the sexual act. Honor the divine within your partner.

Wise Words

Svadhisthana means "abode of the vital force" or "dwelling place of the self."

A healthy second chakra connects us to others without losing our identity.

The desire of this chakra is to create and expand without limitation.

Chakra 3: Manipura

Intention

To awaken and balance the third chakra.

Approximate Length

3 minutes

Lesson

The third chakra, manipura, is located at the navel center, where the body's energy battery is stored. As prana rises from the first and second chakras, it has the potential to become a powerful force in our lives. This chakra is associated with the element of fire and vibrates to the color yellow.

Within this chakra, we develop strength, willpower, and courage. While the second chakra may get you moving to make positive changes, such as quitting smoking or changing jobs, it's the force from the third chakra that enables you to drive through the excursion. The intensity of the navel center is involved in our self-esteem, courage, and the power of transformation.

When this chakra is balanced, we're able to take risks, we feel a sense of inner power and self-confidence, and we are able to make lasting changes. When this chakra is lacking, we have little energy, bad digestion, low self-esteem, and we often feel intimidated. If this chakra is extreme, we're controlling, competitive, stubborn, and we put too much emphasis on power and social status.

Ulcers, chronic fatigue, and digestive problems are common third-chakra ailments.

Today our practice for opening and balancing the manipura chakra embraces poses that fan the flames of the inner fire. In an effort to nourish this chakra on its dynamic journey, it's important for the body's center of gravity to have good muscle tone. This supports posture and promotes a sense of power and determination. Having good muscle tone in the abdomen also enhances all the yoga postures, and it strengthens every system in the body.

Our inner focus is on moving with will and purpose, on energizing limbs and torso, and on building and storing prana.

Asanas for Deepening

Begin with navasana (low reclining boat). Keep legs, head, and shoulders about two inches (five centimeters) off the ground and hold the posture for 5 to 10 breaths. Repeat three to five times.

Perform paschimottanasana (posterior stretch) with a chant. *Ram* is the seed sound of the third chakra. As you exhale into posterior stretch, audibly say, "Ram." Hold your awareness at the navel through your exhale. Repeat three times.

Uddiyana bandha (stomach lift) takes energy from the first and second chakras and moves it up to the third chakra for the purpose of purifying and detoxifying the system. From a standing position, bend forward and rest your hands just above your knees. Exhale completely, pulling your belly back toward the spine. Apply mula bandha (root lock). Lift the lower abdomen upward under the rib cavity so that the navel center appears concave. Drop the chin toward the chest. Hold. When you need to inhale, lift the chin and release the belly and mula bandha. Repeat three times.

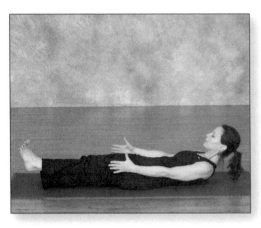

Navasana

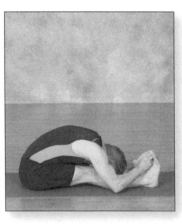

Paschimottanasana

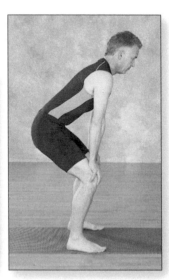

Uddiyana bandha

Standing strength flow. This series warms the body and builds strength in the abdomen one side at a time. Feel the warrior energy, and move from the navel center in all postures. Take five breaths in each asana before moving to the next.

1. Tadasana (mountain pose, photo *a*).
2. Virabhadrasana I (warrior I, photo *b*).
3. Parshvottanasana (angle, photo *c*).
4. Virabhadrasana II (warrior II, photo *d*).
5. Trikonasana (triangle, photo *e*).
6. Parshvakonasana (triangle II, photo *f*) with arm wrap (binding).
7. Adho mukha shvanasana (down dog, photo *g*).
8. Tadasana (mountain pose, photo *h*).

Standing Strength Flow

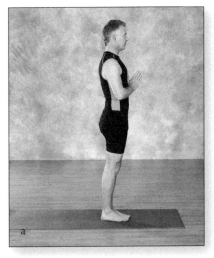

Tadasana

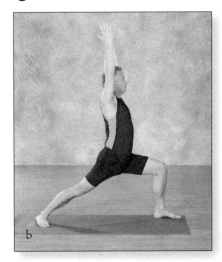

Virabhadrasana I

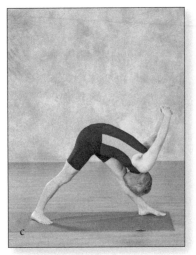

Parshvottanasana

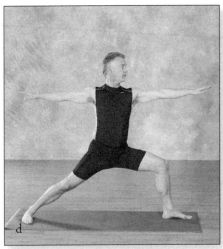

Virabhadrasana II

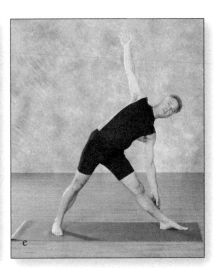

Trikonasana

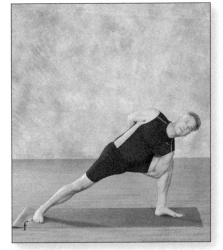

Parshvakonasana

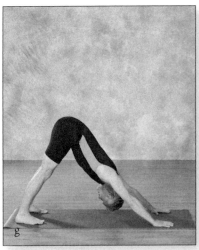

Adho mukha shvanasana

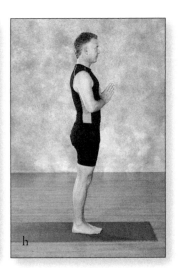

Tadasana

Practice Off the Mat

Risk it. Move beyond what feels safe. Gently push yourself into something new. Start small. For some, taking a risk may mean asking the waiter for more mayonnaise. For others, it's buying a house. Weigh the risk in relation to what seems appropriate for the health of your third chakra.

Make a list of daily goals, and use your will to accomplish each one. For change to take place and for new habits to be made, don't overwhelm yourself with goals. Start small. One item may simply be to make your bed each morning.

Wise Words

Manipura means "jewel of the lotus" or "lustrous gem."

A balanced third chakra connects us with our internal source of power and with the body's energy battery.

Chakra 4: Anahata

Intention

To awaken and balance the heart center.

Approximate Length

3 minutes

Lesson

The fourth chakra, or heart center, is the center of the chakra system. Its physical location is the heart, lungs, thymus gland, upper chest, upper back, shoulders, arms, and hands. The heart chakra vibrates to the color emerald green, and its element is air, which spreads and energizes.

This chakra is the balance point between the lower three chakras and the upper three chakras. It lies halfway between Mother Earth, our connection to the physical plane, and Father Sky, our connection to the spiritual plane. The heart center integrates the two.

This chakra carries the seed of inner peace and harmony, and as the center expands, the seed opens and grows. When this chakra is balanced, we are able to give and receive love; we are caring, compassionate, accepting, and we have a peaceful spirit. When the heart is lacking, we have feelings of shyness and loneliness, an inability to forgive, a lack of empathy; we're critical, intolerant, and resentful. If you notice that your shoulders are rounded inward and your heart sunken, it may be difficult to feel the physical movement that enables the emotional journey to begin.

Symptoms of an overactive fourth chakra include codependency, jealousy, and possessiveness. We've all known people who were jealous of our friends or relatives, or those who felt a certain ownership of the relationship.

Physical imbalances manifest as shallow breathing, asthma, high blood pressure, and heart disease.

Our yoga practices for opening the heart chakra involve working with the supporting anatomy around the heart in order to give the chest some breathing room. Our internal focus is on releasing blocked or overflooded emotion. We'll lead with the heart center, working from the heart, not from the head.

Asanas for Deepening

In breathing bhujangasana (cobra), breathe in and out of the pose. Open to sensation with each inhale, maintaining that opening as you release to the floor with each exhale.

The heart center naturally desires to release and let go. Doing backbends, such as dhanurasana (bow), develops the physical expansion and surrender we need in order to open the heart completely.

Trikonasana (triangle) is lovingly referred to as "the posture of joy" because of its heart-opening capabilities. Make sure to spread the wings of the shoulders, and feel the heart's backdoor expand between the blades.

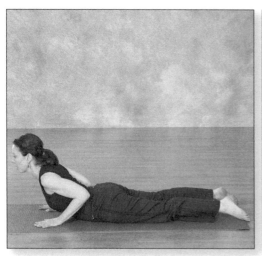

Bhujangasana

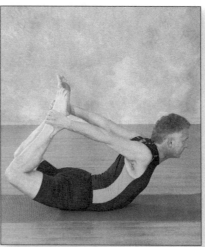

Dhanurasana

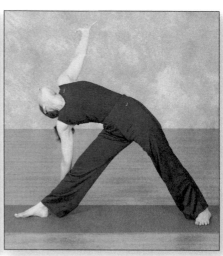

Trikonasana

Heart-opening vinyasa. In heart-opening vinyasa, emphasize broadening the shoulders, opening the chest, lifting the sternum, and expanding the supporting anatomy around the heart. Hold each position for five breaths.

1. Easy pose with side stretch (photo *a*).
2. Easy pose twist (photo *b*).
3. Seated yoga mudra with hands interlaced behind the back (photo *c*). Bring forehead to the ground.
4. Adho mukha shvanasana (down dog, photo *d*) to urdhva mukha shvanasana (up dog, photo *e*) to adho mukha shvanasana (down dog, photo *f*).
5. Standing yoga mudra (photo *g*).
6. Tadasana (mountain pose) with hands in namaste (photo *h*). Tune in to the rhythm of the heartbeat.

Heart-Opening Vinyasa

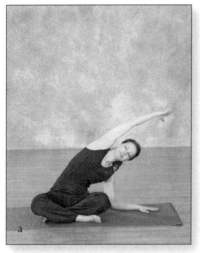

Easy pose with side stretch

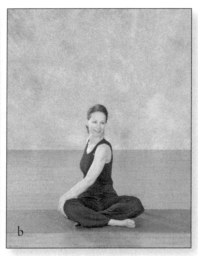

Easy pose twist

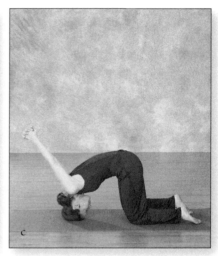

Seated yoga mudra

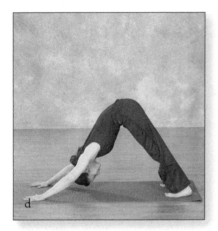

Adho mukha shvanasana

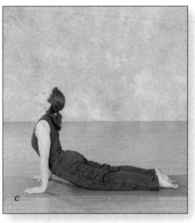

Urdhva mukha shvanasana

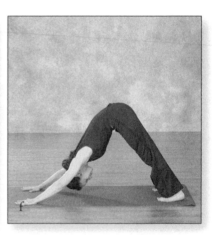

Adho mukha shvanasana

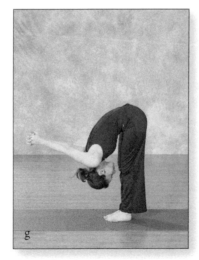

Standing yoga mudra

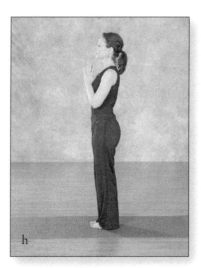

Tadasana

Heart connection. Anahata governs the sense of touch and rules the hands. Bring the hands together in namaste (anjali mudra) and experience the sensation of hand touching hand. This completes the energy circuit between the hands and the heart and harmonizes the two hemispheres of the brain. Focus the awareness on anahata chakra. Silently chant, "Yam," the seed sound of the heart, with each exhale. Feel the vibration gently stirring the heart center.

Practice Off the Mat

Practice gratitude. Gratitude invites the heart to open. Realize how much we have to be thankful for. Thank your loved ones, neighbors, and coworkers. Keep a gratitude journal. Every day, write down five things that you are grateful for.

Give of yourself. Call someone who is lonely; spend time with others who need companionship; do a favor for someone without expecting anything in return.

Forgive. Forgiveness is essential for a healthy heart chakra. It frees the heart so that energy can move forward. Forgiveness doesn't mean you forget or that you even have to involve the other person. It's simply a method to accept the past, to get on with your life, and to get your heart energy moving.

Wise Words

When fear or depression sets into the body, the body contracts in an effort to defend itself.

The heart chakra connects the heart to our hands. What the hands are engaged in directly impacts the heart, and what the heart feels impacts the hands.

Anahata means unstuck, fresh, clean, unhurt.

When the heart is balanced, we are open to the vibrations of universal love.

The life force of the heart connects us to a higher spiritual power, our own heart, and the hearts of others.

Chakra 5: Visuddha

Intention

To identify and balance the throat-center chakra.

Approximate Length

2 minutes

Lesson

The fifth chakra, the throat center, is the first chakra that is primarily focused on the spiritual plane. It is associated with the color blue and the element of sound. Vibration, rhythm, music, voice, words, and communication are associated with this center. Music, dancing, singing, and communicating through writing and speaking are all fifth-chakra ways to express ourselves.

When this chakra is balanced, we become aware of the world on the level of vibration, and we are in tune with our surroundings. The voice is full, listening skills are good, and there are few miscommunications.

When energy is lacking in the throat, we have difficulty putting feelings into words, we fear speaking, we speak in a soft voice, and we often have secrets. Those with an overactive throat center tend to talk too much and too loudly; they also gossip, criticize, and are unable to listen.

Physical imbalances may manifest as neck stiffness, teeth grinding, jaw disorders, throat ailments, or as an underactive or overactive thyroid.

Our asana practice for opening this chakra includes moving with sound, letting sound move the body, and using sound to release blockages.

Asanas for Deepening

Select any posture, such as standing sidebend or parshvottanasana (angle), and say, "Ham" (pronounced "hum") on each exhale. *Ham* is the seed sound of the throat chakra.

Perform neck rolls. Turn the head from side to side, and bring the ear to the shoulder using the seed sound *ham* on the exhale.

In halasana (plow), extend from the buttocks to the heels. Relax the brain. Keep an opening between your chin and sternum. This helps stimulate the thyroid gland.

Bhramari breath is the sound of the bumblebee. It clears the mind, soothes the nervous system, and stimulates the throat center. Simulate the drone of a bumblebee on the exhale.

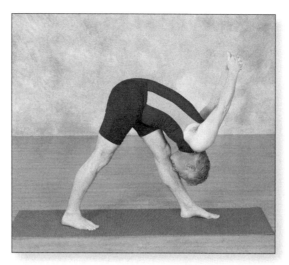

Parshvottanasana

Neck Rolls

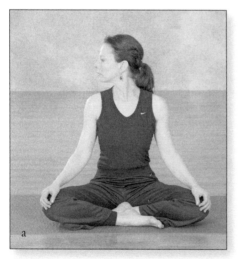

Look over shoulder

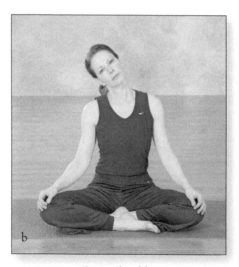

Ear to shoulder

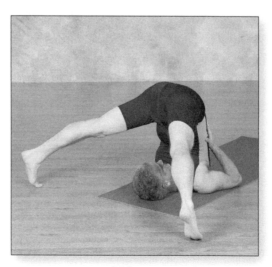

Halasana

Practice Off the Mat

Listen. For one day, *really* listen to the people around you. Give others your full attention when they speak to you, and show interest and enthusiasm in what they are saying—and don't interrupt!

Make no complaints. Avoid criticizing anyone or complaining about anything for one day. This especially includes criticizing yourself. Enjoy the freedom from negative energies.

Try peppermint. Add one drop of peppermint essential oil to a glass of water to help open up expression. The peppermint cleanses the throat of mucus and helps clear away psychic debris.

Use a mantra meditation. Mantra is a tool of the mind that protects us from the traps of nonproductive thought and action. The rhythm of the sound works on a subconscious level. It penetrates our conscious thoughts by affecting their rhythm. If you don't have a mantra, take a moment to sit quietly each day and say a daily affirmation to yourself. It can be a personal goal or a wish for a loved one. When you say it every day, it becomes a part of you. If you believe this affirmation, you'll become connected to it and it to you.

Wise Words

Visuddha means purification. The release of sound purifies and organizes the energy in the body for entry into higher consciousness.

Sound as a vibration is purifying. Sound affects the cellular structure of matter.

The gift of the throat chakra is to be heard and understood, and to receive truth.

Chakra 6: Ajna

Intention

To awaken and balance the spiritual eye, also called "the third eye."

Approximate Length

3 minutes

Lesson

In the sixth chakra, the spiritual eye, the journey of consciousness moves deeper into our inner world. Here we find the source of our inner light. This center is associated with the element of light and the color indigo. Its location is between and just above the physical eyes.

The sixth chakra is the home of intuition, dreams, and visions. As children, this chakra is open and active. Colors are more vivid. We have imaginary playmates, and we see dragons, witches, and castles. But as we get older, the world forces this energy center to close. As adults, we have to reconnect with this inner window by looking beyond the material world. These internal visual attributes include clairvoyance, telepathy, intuition, dreaming, and visualization.

When this chakra is balanced, intuition, memory, creativity, and dream recall are strong. When this chakra is overactive, we may experience difficulty concentrating and have headaches, hallucinations, and nightmares. If this chakra is closed, memory is poor and visualization capabilities are lacking. We may have an inability to see alternatives and become skeptical.

Our asana focus today is on inviting stillness and openness into our inner window and on imagining the energy from the lower chakras moving up into the spiritual eye.

Asanas for Deepening

Begin this practice with the eye exercises, doing each variation three times. Then, for the following asana practice, gently close your eyes. Keeping the eyes closed during an entire class gives us a fresh perspective on the postures and their healing qualities. Because the eyes provide 85 percent of our sensory input, students won't be distracted by the room, by other students, or by looking critically at their own bodies.

Do each variation of the eye exercises three times.

1. Look center, up, center, down (photo *a*).
2. Move the eyes clockwise in a circle, then counterclockwise (photo *b*).
3. Focus the gaze on something far away, such as on a tree outside the window, then move the gaze to an object that is close, such as the tip of a finger.

Matsyasana (fish) puts the focus directly on the third eye.

For earth-to-eye squat, in squat position, bring the hands to the ground in front of the body. Inhale. Exhale and move your forehead to the ground as energy moves into the third eye. Repeat eight times.

Perform this triangle variation of balasana (child's pose). Place your hands on the floor under the forehead, with your thumbs and index fingers touching, making a triangle where the third eye is. Breathe life force into the spiritual triangle.

In padmasana (lotus), chant, "Om," the seed sound of the spiritual eye, with each exhalation. Rest awareness at the eyebrow center, visualizing energy moving up and down along the subtle channel between the root and eyebrows.

Eye Exercises

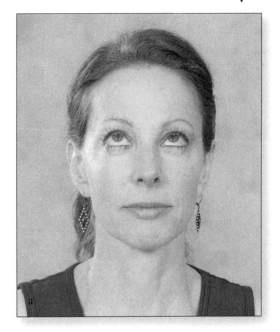

Look center, up, center, down

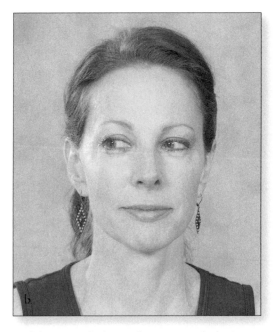

Move eyes clockwise then counterclockwise

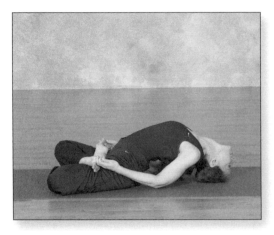

Matsyasana

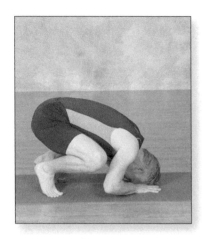

Earth-to-eye squat

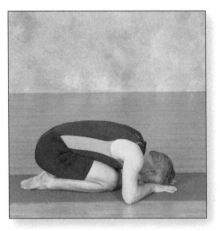

Balasana

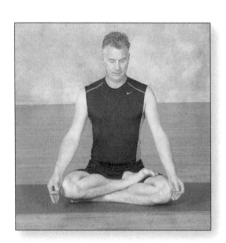

Padmasana

Practice Off the Mat

Light up your life. Light is stimulating to consciousness, and it wakes us up. Light up your home. A dark home can be depressing. Add lamps and open drapes. Buy more mirrors, and light candles in order to shed some light on your third eye.

Keep a dream journal. Buy a dream interpretation dictionary and record your dreams, even if you can remember only bits and pieces. Dreams reveal the dynamics of our subconscious.

Apply tiger balm to the third eye. This helps bring heat and physical awareness to the eyebrow center.

Wise Words

Ajna means command, perception, knowledge, and authority.

The ajna chakra is the window to the soul.

Clairvoyance is not just for the gifted few. We all have the ability see clearly if we look deeper and trust our instincts.

Chakra 7: Sahasrara

Intention

To awaken and balance the crown chakra.

Approximate Length

2 minutes

Lesson

The seventh chakra is located at the top of the head, and it serves as the crown of the chakra system, symbolizing the seat of enlightenment. The element of the seventh chakra is thought, which corresponds with the highest functions of the mind. It vibrates to the color violet.

Development of the other chakras from the root chakra upward is a prerequisite for the goal of moving energy up to the crown. Here we are open to divine intelligence, wisdom, and understanding. We feel oneness with a higher power, knowing there is no separation between it and us.

When the crown chakra is balanced, we feel at peace with ourselves; we have an inner wisdom and a spiritual connection; and we are open-minded. When this chakra is overactive, a person may live in his or her head, have feelings of being a spiritual elitist, or be disassociated from the body. If the crown center is lacking energy, a person may be a spiritual cynic or skeptic, have difficulty thinking, or have a closed mind or rigid belief systems.

Today's asana practice for opening and balancing this chakra is to focus on the awareness of awareness, to witness consciousness, to release attachments, and to connect to a higher power.

Asanas for Deepening

Begin with uttanasana (standing forward bend) to bring blood flow into the crown. Move into chakrasana (wheel), then handstand against the wall. Complete shirshasana (headstand or tripod) and then practice nadi shodhana (alternate-nostril breathing) pranayama. Finish with padmasana (lotus). Chant, "Om," with each exhalation. Rest awareness at the crown center, visualizing energy moving up and down an imaginary channel between the root and the crown.

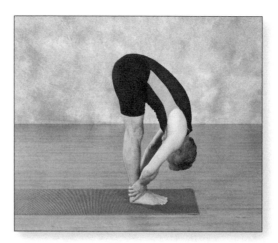

Uttanasana

Chakrasana

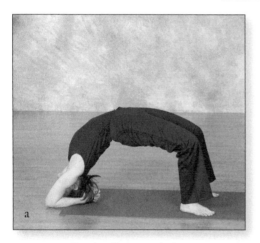

On the elbows variation

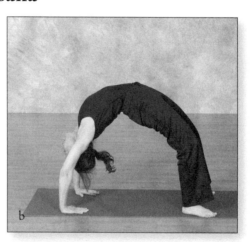

Lifted pose

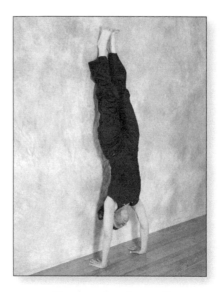

Handstand against wall

Shirshasana

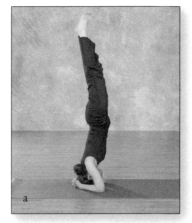

Headstand

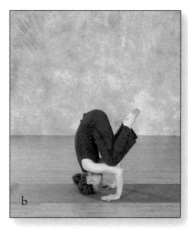

Tripod

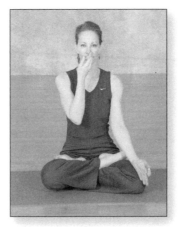

Nadi shodhana

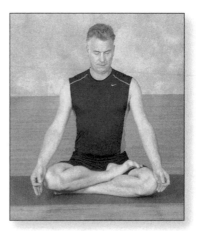

Padmasana

Practice Off the Mat

Honor the divine. Visualize your concept of divine spirit, whether it's God, angels, Jesus, or Buddha. Set time aside each day for spiritual practice and prayer. Look outside and honor the wonder of nature.

The seventh limb in Raja yoga is dhyana, or meditation. Meditation is the optimal yogic practice for bringing the crown chakra into balance. Meditation connects us to divine energy and expanded consciousness, and it empowers the mind to become more present, clear, and insightful. Just as asana has been called "dental floss for the body," meditation is mental floss for the mind.

Wise Words

Sahasrara means "thousand-petal lotus."

The purpose of opening and balancing the crown center is to tune in to and surrender to divine consciousness.

Those who are enlightened know the unknown, and they experience the transcendental meaning of life.

Chakras and the Five Tibetans

Intention

To keep the chakras spinning and learn the Five Tibetan rites.

Approximate Length

30 minutes, including the Five Tibetan practices

Lesson

For thousands of years, holistic practitioners have known that the body has seven principal energy centers—chakras—where the nadis, the body's subtle energy channels, intersect. The chakras, located along the spinal column, are considered transformation centers and are linked to specific areas of the body and mind. These seven energy centers form the major components of our consciousness.

The chakras regulate the flow of prana, or life force. Prana can be released for physical, emotional, or spiritual functions, or it can be held and ultimately blocked, causing disruptions in the body. An accumulation of toxins in the internal organs can also interfere with the flow of prana. When this happens, we may manifest psychological or somatic illnesses. Many of these disharmonies can be treated successfully by readjusting and harmonizing the chakras.

The Five Tibetan rites are a series of exercises that are said to hold the key to lasting youth, health, and vitality because they keep the chakras spinning. Here are some of the benefits of the Five Tibetans:

- They balance the hormones. When all of the endocrine glands are functioning in harmony, we have more energy and more vitality. Balanced hormones also help alleviate PMS and menopausal discomforts.
- They enhance bone mass. The Tibetans are weight-bearing exercises that stress every bone in the body.
- They help drain the lymph system. The lymph system moves toxins out of the body. The actions of the Tibetans, as they compress and stretch the various organs, glands, and muscles, assist in draining the lymph system. The result is that you flush toxins faster.
- They give you energy throughout the day.

The quickest way to regain youth, health, and vitality is to prompt these energy centers into spinning normally again. The Five Tibetans do just that.

It takes about 20 minutes to do the full 21 repetitions of each of these rites. For beginners, it's suggested that you start with three to five repetitions a day for the first week and then increase the number by two repetitions every week until you reach the full 21 repetitions. Today we'll do five repetitions of each.

[Guide students through a brief warm-up such as slow-moving surya namaskara (sun salutation) before introducing the Five Tibetans.]

Asanas for Deepening

Rite 1: Spinning. Stand in mountain pose with arms outstretched, horizontal to the floor. Slowly spin around clockwise. (In the southern hemisphere, spin counterclockwise.) It's normal to feel slightly dizzy.

Rite 2: Leg lift. Lie flat on the floor, face up. Extend your arms along your sides and place the palms of your hands against the floor. Inhale and raise your head off the floor, tucking the chin against the chest. As you do this, lift your legs, knees straight, into a vertical position. If possible, let the legs extend back over the body, toward the head. Exhale and slowly lower both the head and the legs, knees straight, to the floor.

Rite 3: Camel. Kneel on the floor. On the exhale, bring the head and neck forward, tucking the chin against the chest. Then on the inhale, place the hands against the lower back and bring the head and neck back, arching the spine and tucking in the tailbone. Exhale and return to the original position.

Rite 4: Table lift. Sit on the floor with your legs straight out in front of you and your feet about 12 inches (about 30 centimeters) apart. Place the palms of your hands on the floor alongside the hips. Tuck the chin against the chest. Inhale and gently bring the head back as far as it will go. At the same time, raise your body so that the knees bend, tracking straight ahead toward the top of the feet, while the arms remain straight. The trunk of the body should be horizontal to the floor, in a straight line with the upper legs. Tense every muscle in the body. Exhale and relax your muscles as you return to the original sitting position.

Rite 5: Updog and downdog. Lie face down. Place your palms on the floor beneath your shoulders and turn the toes under. Inhale and lift your head, neck, and chest so that your arms are perpendicular to the floor and the spine is arched, pelvis lifted so that the body is in a sagging position and the legs are off the ground (updog). Exhale and bend at the hips. Stay up high on the toes. Bring the body up into an inverted V. At the same time, bring the chin forward, tucking it against the chest (downdog).

Relax in shavasana for five minutes.

Rite 1: Spinning

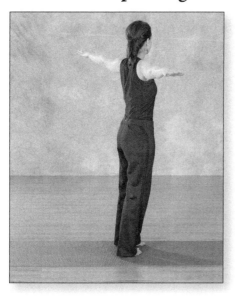

Rite 2: Leg Lift

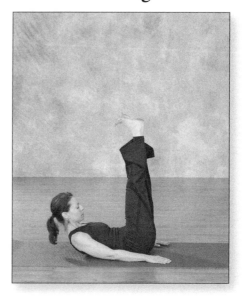

Rite 3: Camel

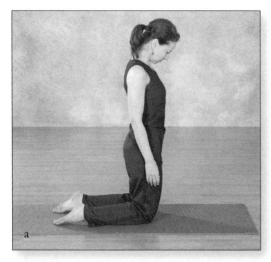

Head down

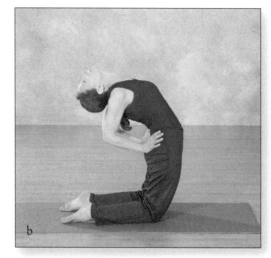

Head back

Rite 4: Table Lift

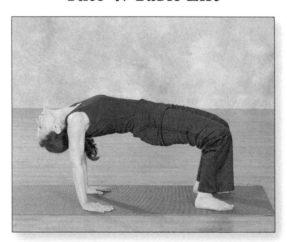

Rite 5: Updog and Downdog

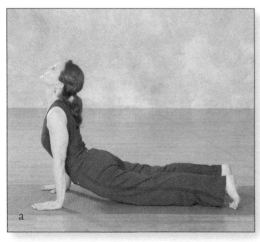

Updog

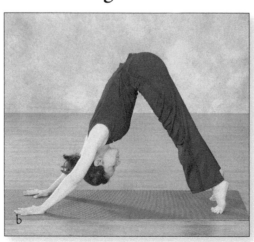

Downdog

Practice Off the Mat

Practice the Five Tibetans every day for a week. Notice a welcome increase in energy levels, with vitality lasting through the day. Many people reduce or stop their coffee consumption completely once starting the practice. Avoid practicing the Five Tibetans two to three hours before bedtime.

Wise Words

The symptoms of old age and physical degeneration set in when the chakras slow down.

Chant, "Om," which vibrates and awakens all the chakras.

The chakras are like traffic circles, with the nadis connecting to each chakra.

Chapter 12
Lessons of the Heart Center

Teach this triple truth to all: A generous heart, kind speech, and a life of service and compassion are the things that renew humanity.

—**Buddha**

The heart is the temple of the soul. The heart holds the secrets to self-knowledge. Unlike the brain, the heart center doesn't use words to express itself; rather the heart is about sensation, feeling, and emotion. To know something by heart suggests that it comes from within, without the energy of thought.

Every one of us prospers within our heart's love embrace. Love is both the source and the seed that bring life. Here the most important lessons of our existence are identified, digested, and assimilated into our consciousness.

When we connect with our heart through our yoga practice, the transformational powers of yoga extend beyond ourselves. They extend out into the universe.

Anjali Mudra: Namaste

Intention

To learn the meaning behind the gesture of namaste.

Approximate Time

5 minutes

Lesson

At the beginning or end of a yoga class, we bring our hands together while saying "Namaste," which translates to, "The light in me bows to the light in you." This salutation is the nucleus of our practice, of seeing the light within all of creation. The hand position is called anjali mudra.

Anjali comes from the Sanskrit root *anj*, meaning "to honor or celebrate." Mudra means "seal." We find this hand gesture within certain asanas, such as tadasana at the beginning and end of sun salutations, in warrior I with our hands over our head or on our chest, or in balance poses such as tree.

As we bring our hands together at the center, we are connecting the right and left hemispheres of the brain. This is the yogic process of yoking or uniting our active and receptive natures, right and left sides, masculine and feminine energies, logic and intuition, sun and moon, and the strengths and weaknesses of our dual nature. It has been said that the right hand represents our higher self or the divine, while the left hand represents the lower, worldly nature.

Let's begin by coming into sukhasana (easy pose), sitting high on the pelvic bones. Lengthen your spine out of your pelvis, broaden your shoulder blades in order to spread your chest open from the inside. Lift up through your crown, and extend the back of your neck by dropping your chin slightly. Be aware of energy rising up from your tailbone as you follow your breath to the crown. Inhale and reach further. Broaden your ribs and listen to your breath until there is no breath left to inhale, and then exhale until there is no breath left to exhale. On the next inhalation, cross your legs the opposite way.

Now, with open palms, lift the arms out to the sides, extending your heart center. Slowly, mindfully, draw your hands together at the center of your chest, gathering all your vitality into your heart. Consciously notice how both sides of our nature are connected here at the heart. Acknowledge how this centered inner-state inspires today's practice.

Asanas for Deepening

Anjali mudra can be used within many other asanas as a way to come back to and maintain your center. As you bring your hands together, ground your intentions within your heart.

During sun salutation (see pages 58-59), practice anjali mudra at the beginning, at the end, and during the lunge sequence, adding a twist with the back knee off the ground in runner's stretch.

In virabhadrasana I (warrior I), bring the hands together overhead.

In vrikshasana (tree), merge with the earth energy through an upward movement into the heart and above.

During matsyasana (fish in butterfly variation), feel the spiritual interface between the pelvic center and the heart and between the heart and the crown chakra.

Finally, in navasana (boat), see if you can identify the heat of transformation and will that comes from the navel center along with the wisdom of the heart.

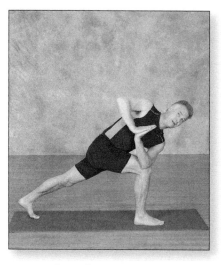
Sun salutation variation

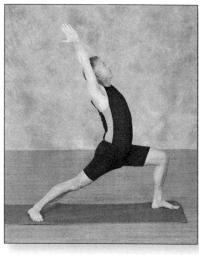
Virabhadrasana I

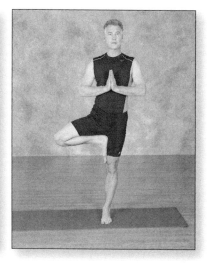
Vrikshasana

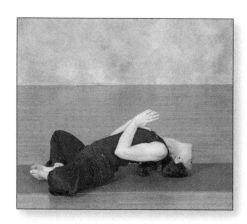
Matsyasana

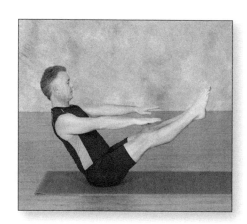
Navasana

Practice Off the Mat

Anjali mudra is used as a posture of composure, to communicate our heartfelt energy, whether we are meeting someone for the first time or saying goodbye. Anjali mudra is bestowed to teachers, family, friends, students, and strangers. It is a humbling gesture given to nature and deities, and it is offered at meals.

Wise Words

In yoga philosophy, the energetic heart is visualized as a lotus at the center of the chest. Anjali mudra acknowledges this lotus heart, directing it to open to the light.

Anjali mudra is an asana, balancing and harmonizing our energies, keeping us centered, clear, and positive.

Feel the heart come alive, and beam with the glow of harmony that is within you.

Seeds of Love

Intention

To scatter and plant our seeds of love.

Approximate Time

3 to 4 minutes

Lesson

To plant or spread the seeds of love is one of the main themes of yoga practice. It's important to remember this during your practice so that the heart and mind can unite. When we bring our love to everything we do, we make each conscious thought a compassionate thought.

We practice yoga so that we can truly experience the heart center by tapping first into the physical attributes of the heart and then into the subtle energies of this connector of our physical and spiritual beings.

Think of spreading the seeds of love this way: Just as one drop can spread ripples through an entire body of water, the love we give or visualize can send a sacred ripple out that will be felt by the collective consciousness.

Let's put our hands in anjali mudra. Breathe into the heart and visualize the seeds of love that you spread out into your world. Now bring your hands to your lap, separate your palms, and open your hands to resemble the bud of a lotus flower. Using your heart-and-mind connection, plant a love-seed prayer or affirmation, such as "peace," "clarity," or "good health" within your opened anjali mudra flower. Drop your chin and visualize the manifestation of your prayer. Let's begin our asana practice with a newly awakened sense of humility and respect.

Asanas for Deepening

During uttanasana (forward bend), surrender to the earth's love.

While practicing adho mukha shvanasana (downward dog), drop the head below the heart.

For tabletop twist, lean on one arm and lift the opposite arm.

While in bharaduajasana (half-lotus bound twist), squeeze the heart and release the nourished seeds of love.

For dwi pada viparita dandasana (bridge variation), interlace your hands behind your neck and lift the heart from the diaphragm, moving the crown of the head to the floor.

For dhanurasana (side bow), roll from bow to side bow, leading with each side of the heart. Finish with a lunge with backbend.

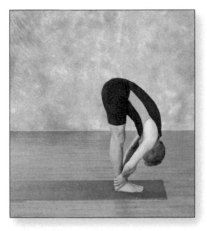

Uttanasana

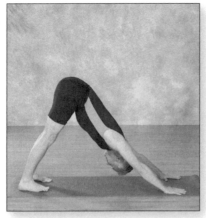

Adho mukha shvanasana

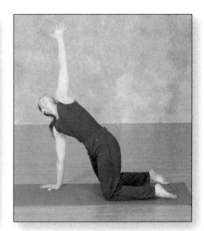

Tabletop twist

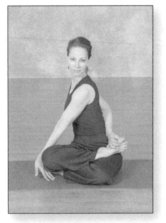

Bharaduajasana

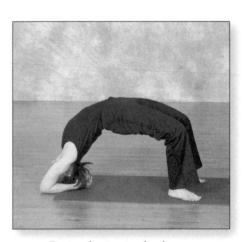

Dwi pada viparita dandasana

Dhanurasana

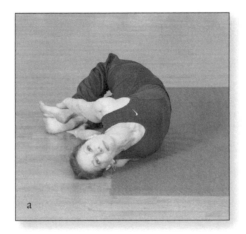

a

Roll onto right side

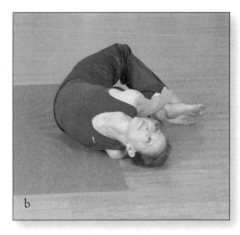

b

Roll onto left side

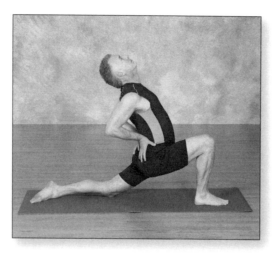

Lunge with backbend

Practice Off the Mat

There are countless ways to spread the seeds of love. Here are a few examples:

- Send a note or e-mail of gratitude and appreciation to a coworker for a job well-done.
- Look into the eyes of each person you interact with in an effort to look into his or her heart and soul. Then transmit compassion and love through a sincere smile.
- Plant some flower seeds. When they bloom, pick some and give a bouquet to someone you love.
- Every time you take out the trash, give thanks for all the goods, services, and blessings you received from each item before it became trash.

Wise Words

The soul vibrates from the heart. Our vibrations get smoother and steadier as we become more in-touch with the heart.

As you focus on the heart, imagine it as emerald green, and experience its virtues as it fills your entire being with love.

Living in appreciation makes every day a blessing.

Expanding the Heart

Intention

To expand the wisdom of the heart center.

Approximate Time

5 minutes

Lesson

We've heard about the power of positive thinking, that we are what we think. If we think positive thoughts, we become positive. If we think kind thoughts, we become kind. If we are negative and bitter, we become that as well.

When we shift our feelings to positive, loving emotions, our heart rhythms immediately shift. This change creates a series of physiological events that assist the whole body: Blood pressure normalizes, stress hormones drop, and our immune system gets a boost. Even anti-aging hormones increase, suggesting that negative thinking has an influence on how we age.

So much of what we do in asana practice requires awareness and an opening of the heart center. Let's begin this awareness practice with a simple exercise that opens the delicate passages of the heart chakra and allows us to have compassion for those in our lives.

Stay in your seated position and close your eyes. Place your right hand over your heart and your left hand below your navel. Spreading your fingers, breathe into your left hand and let the right hand feel the warmth coming from your heart. Bring the breath down and let the energy rise up from the root into the heart.

Stay here with your eyes closed and your jaw relaxed. Let yourself feel the vibrations in your body, in and out, and the light above and between the eyebrows. Visualize your breathing going in and out through the area of your heart. Now focus on someone whom you have gratitude for—your spouse, children, friends—as well as the many good things you have in your life such as your home, job, and the food you eat. Send them admiration, wisdom, and compassion as you continue to breathe in and out through your heart.

Sense a white light above your head that is filled with peace and love. Visualize this light coming into the crown of your head and gathering in the heart center. Explore the emotion of love arising within. Now send the same emotions of compassion and love to yourself as we begin our asana practice.

Asanas for Deepening

The following asanas are utilized for expanding the area around the physical heart and lungs. Feel the stretch from side to side and up and down. Focus your intentions on expanding the wisdom of the sacred heart. Discover the calm that resides within. Use the internal chant *om mani padme hum*, which means "The wisdom of the jewel of the lotus resides in my heart," as you move through the asanas.

For natarajasana (king dancer) variation, stand with your heel to your sit bones. Press the heel toward the pelvic bone as you lightly arch back.

For setu bandha sarvangasana (bridge), wall variation, utilize the wall as a dynamic, inverted support system for heart expansion.

Sarvanga padmasana (shoulderstand lotus) opens the hips in an effort to release positive energy. Feel the prana flow into the heart from the pelvis.

In parighasana (gate), lengthen both sides of the waist and stretch the side ribs.

Finally, in prasarita padottanasana (spread-leg forward bend), feel the heart energy working toward the throat center.

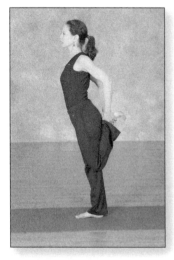
Natarajasana variation

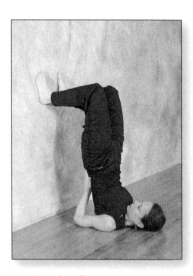
Setu bandha sarvangasana

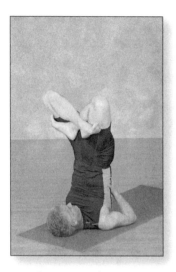
Sarvanga padmasana

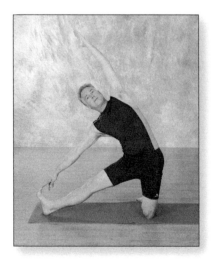
Parighasana

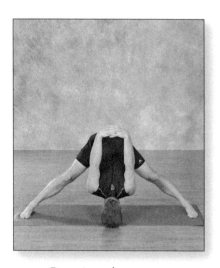
Prasarita padottanasana

Practice Off the Mat

Today's experiences may be setting the groundwork for future healing. The more you release negative emotions as you speak, act, and talk, the more positive free-flowing energy, light, and laughter will flourish within.

Wise Words

Remember the opportunities that are born of love.

Find out what you are willing to welcome into your heart, not just into your physical practice, but into your life.

When you practice asana, do it through your heart rather than through the brain's anatomical-alignment instructions. Recognize how that changes the flow of prana.

Reversing Negative Emotion

Intention

To discover the yogic methods that help us work through and release negative emotion.

Approximate Time

5 to 7 minutes

Lesson

When we experience very intense negative emotions, the simple act of staying present through the experience can lead us to a place of spaciousness, change, and growth. Sitting with the energy of negative emotions, including the situations and negative baggage that may be at the root of them, is the exact opposite of avoiding them, trying to make them go away, or hoping a magic pill will destroy them. Our yoga practice teaches us that none of these options are effective means of healing ourselves.

Quieting the mind and sustaining a solid connection with the heart—locking into its power—reverses the stress effects of negative emotion. This can be accomplished by breathing through your heart in times of stress and crisis with the intention of consciously easing the emotions of sadness, anxiety, and fear.

Take a moment right now to listen to your thoughts. When we have the strength to get close to our negative emotions—conversations that went on, hurtful incidents we're holding on to—without getting caught up in our reactions to them, they lose their force. It's important to know that our positive and loving energy is much more powerful than that of the negative energy.

To practice, bring negative emotion into your heart. Hold the feeling there. It helps to say to yourself, "I'm feeling angry," or, "I'm sad," or, "I'm afraid." Focus on your breathing, following your breath as it moves in and out through your nostrils. Let your heart space expand until you have the sensation that there is real space around your feeling. Now notice what happens, how the excessive activity shifts. Your sadness or anger might become sharper for a while, or it might begin to soften and become less annoying. Feel where it is in your body. Some of us feel it between the shoulder blades, behind the heart. Others notice it in the pit of the stomach. Stay present to any color or texture around your mood. If you sense that something needs to be done with this situation, be aware of this but don't get caught up in it. You can go back to it later.

As we sit with our negative emotions, we are shifting our perspective on them. Our intention is to explore the energy of these emotions and to notice how much power we decide to give them.

And now, through asana, let's work out the physical sensations of negative emotions.

Asanas for Deepening

The inner strength it takes to turn upside down helps shake out negative experiences. Try a variation of adho mukha shvanasana (downward dog) on the wall using the half handstand variation (photo *a*). In another variation of adho mukha shvanasana, downward dog is combined with half lotus (photo *b*). The downward inversion, coupled with the hip opening of the half lotus, acts as an elixir for negative emotions.

During parshvottanasana (angle with cow's face arms), stretch through the heart center and deep into the hamstrings.

For the standing backbend against the wall, begin by standing with your back to a wall. Bend backward and walk your hands down the wall to the floor behind you. Envision yourself being daring enough to go into the unknown of what's behind you.

Finish with a virasana (hero) variation. Lean all the way back until your head is on the ground, hands in anjali mudra. Note: Do not lean all the way back if you experience pain in the knees.

Adho Mukha Shvanasana

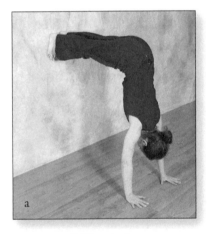

Wall variation

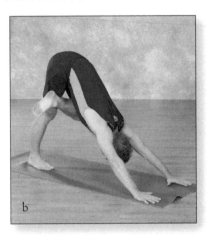

Variation with half lotus

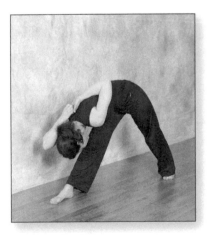

Parshvottanasana

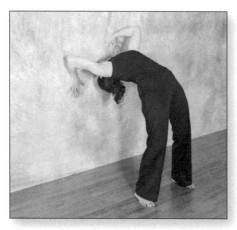
Standing backbend against wall

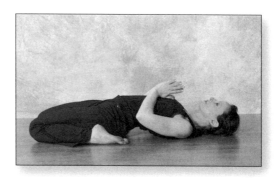
Virasana

Pranayama for anxiety. The anuloma krama breath expands the chest and deepens the inhalation. It's ideal for replacing the energy that is taken by sadness and fear. It also builds inner confidence and thus lifts depression. Please refer to page 90 for instructions.

Practice Off the Mat

While you are going through a healing process, have compassion for yourself. Self-compassion helps reduce nervous system overload.

An important part of emotional healing is bringing your attention into the pain itself and looking into your heart space.

When we experience strong emotions, we often lose touch with our physical bodies. The body may become heavy or full of pain. To become grounded inside your body, feel its foundation, where your body comes in contact with the ground. Bring your attention to the sensation of your feet on the ground; if you're sitting, feel the contact between your buttocks and the cushion or floor.

Wise Words

Through asana, we put the body in a position to explore and change our consciousness.

Our most uncomfortable feelings—anger, sadness, fear, grief—will lead us into a very dark space if we don't know how to distill them, learn from them, and return to our true essence.

How you view the world today can make or break your mood, your relationships, your life.

Choosing to forgive means choosing to alleviate yourself of an unhealthy burden in order to be free of the past.

If we harbor bitterness in our hearts against anyone, we only hurt ourselves. Buddha said, "Holding on to anger is like grasping a hot coal with the intent of throwing it at someone else; you are the one who gets burned."

Chapter 13
Relaxation

Better than a thousand hollow words is one word that brings peace.

—Buddha

Shavasana, the corpse pose, gives us an extraordinary opportunity to clean, clear, and start anew. The practice of shavasana is the yogic way of letting unwanted elements within us die, empowering us to surrender to life. The mirror to the soul gets polished, the heart opens, and our inner teacher awakens. But its more subtle and profound payoff is the experience of relaxation in everything we do. A relaxed consciousness permits us to fully live moment-to-moment experiences. Ironically, being a corpse is the yogi's quintessential wake-up call.

In this chapter, we cover a variety of methods of letting go of negative patterns of consciousness and semi-consciousness. You may discover through the practice of shavasana that the "normal" feelings you have are actually tension that you've become used to. The relaxation lessons ask you to practice only one asana—shavasana—for all the other practices of asana have prepared us for this last and most important one.

Shavasana Variations

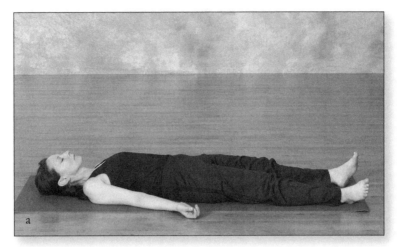

Basic pose

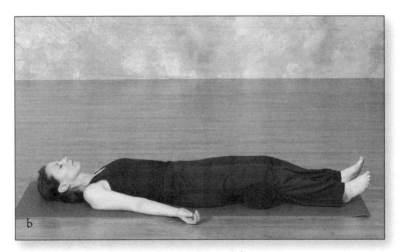

Towel or mat beneath knees

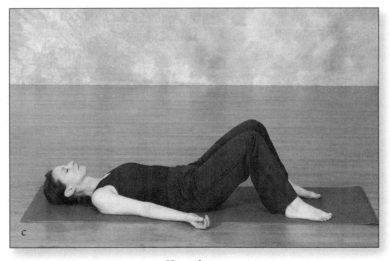

Knees bent

Be a Corpse

Intention

To practice releasing the toxins of the body, mind, and spirit that rise to the surface during asana practice.

Approximate Time

10 minutes

Lesson

Lie in shavasana (corpse pose). As part of our daily sadhana (spiritual practice), shavasana, like many Eastern practices, is a way of preparing for death. This includes the death of the body as well as the surrender of ego attachment, negative emotions, and physical disease, all of which may become dislodged during asana practice.

Gently close your eyes. Rock the head from side to side. Separate your feet about 8 to 10 inches (about 25 centimeters) apart. The palms face upward; fingers are naturally curled.

Make yourself as comfortable as possible and remain in this position unless you begin to experience real discomfort. Constant adjusting or fidgeting will prevent you from experiencing the effects of deep relaxation. If you have any discomfort in your lower back area, place a rolled towel beneath your knees or keep your knees bent, feet flat on the mat.

Allow your attention to be on your smooth, slow, serene flow of breath. The exhale is cleansing and relaxing. The inhale is nourishing and energizing. Turn your attention inward and begin to consider the elements in your body, mind, and spirit that you would like to put to death. Perhaps it's an incident that happened at work, a chronic pain in the shoulder, a worry about someone your love, anything at this moment that you'd like to let go of.

Mentally scan your body from head to toe and back again, pausing briefly to become aware of each area and to release any tension you feel there. Go slowly; tension is habitual, and we don't always recognize when we are holding on to it. You may sense it as a static pull, darkness, or numbness. When you discover tension, imagine sending the breath to that precise part of the body.

Honor the areas that need extra healing. Pause on certain body parts longer if you have pain, limitation, or emotional injury. Remember, this is a practice for living a fuller life, and in order to do that, we need to let certain things die. Clear your mind of the past and the future. When it wanders, simply bring it back to the breath.

The whole body is soft, heavy, and easy. Let it feel like you're melting into the earth. With each exhalation, feel the tension leaving your body, releasing all the body's toxins, wastes, and negative energy. Make your inhalation deep, soothing, and peaceful. Feel the space inside and around your body as tension evaporates.

Relax the crown of your head and the brain, allowing both sides of your brain to release to the floor. Relax your forehead, eyebrows, eyes, eye sockets, and the space between the eyebrows—the mind's eye—and your cheeks and chin. Soften the temples, the jaw, and your neck and throat center.

Relax from the shoulder joints down to the elbows, wrists, and fingertips. Feel the energy in the palms of your hands, and let the movement of your breathing loosen the shoulder blades, mid-back, and lower back. Let the wide muscles of the back release to the ground completely, letting go over and over again through the breath.

Soften the heart center, rib cage, abdominal organs, and pelvis. With a long, slow, deep exhale, recognize the sensation of toxins leaving you. With a long, slow, deep inhale, accept the prana entering your consciousness.

Soften the hips in and around their sockets, then breathe all the way down the thighs, knees, calves, ankles, feet, toes, tips of the toes, and soles of your feet. Continue releasing with your breath until there are no blockages left to explore.

Exhale as though you are breathing from the top of the head down to the tips of the toes. Inhale as though you are breathing from the tips of the toes up to the top of the head. You are now washed in healing light, and you are able to draw everything you need to you. This goodness and healing energy seeps into your body, filling you with a generous, boundless energy and a sense of well-being. Feel it move through the layers of your body, deeper and deeper into every organ, all the way down to the bone.

Experience it in every cell, dissolving any barriers, correcting imbalances.

Now it's just you and your mind. Completely detach yourself from your thoughts, and receive the serenity of the pose and the flow of the moment.

Remain here several minutes, being cautious not to drift off to sleep. [Consider a 5- to 10-minute period of silence at this point.] When you're ready to come out, gently wiggle your fingers and toes. Rock your head from side to side. Roll your body over to one side. Take your top hand and lift yourself up to a seated position. Sit tall, feeling happy and energetic. Be grateful for what you have experienced. Notice your tranquil state of mind, but don't let it end there. Make a commitment to take this feeling with you as you move through your day with joy, serenity, and kindness.

Practice Off the Mat

When the mind feels overwhelmed with drama or worry, stop and pause. Take a moment to visualize how it feels to be in shavasana, mind clear, present, and tuned into the flow of your energy.

Several times during the day, scan your body and notice if you're holding tension. Then let it go.

The practice of relaxation doesn't have to be on the ground. If you need a refresher while at work, practice shavasana in a chair. Gently close your eyes and keep your head, neck and truck in alignment. Take 5 to 10 minutes for a body scan of tension, clearing and quieting the mind.

Palms to the legs. Methodical practices for being present and relaxed can be accomplished almost anywhere. Bring the palms to rest on your thighs and watch the breath. When the mind wanders to thoughts of the past, gently tap your left leg. When the mind wanders off to thoughts of the future, gently tap your right leg. Whenever a thought arises, mentally note *memory* or *fantasy*, then return to the breath.

Wise Words

Give yourself permission to relax. If negative emotions take over, remind yourself that what you're doing now works counter to anxiety and exhaustion.

Practice relaxation as you'd practice asana: with joy, devotion, and an inquiring mind.

If you're busy and want to speed things up, try slowing down first. Slowing down gives you the opportunity to prioritize and tackle the most important work at hand.

It's easy to lose sight of your main purpose amid the distractions of a frenzied mind. Relaxation is cumulative. The more you practice, the better you get at it.

Expanding the Light

Intention

To draw energy from our inner light.

Approximate Time

8 to 10 minutes

Lesson

Please lie in shavasana (corpse pose). Close your eyes and focus on each part of the body. Start from the feet and work your mind upward. Progressively relax until you reach the crown of the head. Give special attention to stiff or painful areas.

Imagine a ball of white light drifting 6 inches (15 centimeters) above your head. The white light is very bright, clear, and it is filled with the most phenomenal, rejuvenating power that you have ever experienced. Feel its energy as it floats above your head. Open your crown chakra and let it receive the gift from this ball of white light. You are completely relaxed, at ease, and wide awake.

Draw down this white-light energy into your forehead, eyes, nose, cheeks, and chin. Draw down this white-light energy into your throat, shoulders, elbows, wrists, and hands. Feel it in your fingertips; feel them tingle. Draw down the white-light energy into your chest, hips, thighs, knees, calves, ankles, and into each toe. Feel the toes tingle as this light fills them. Visualize this light filling your entire body.

Now expand this white light to include the entire room. Breathe healing energy and love into it. Feel yourself expanding, your light going out further and further until it shines through the whole room, then further until it shines through the whole building and whole town. Feel yourself as the light breaks through the darkness and shines out in every direction. Finally, broaden the light to reach all the people who are a part of your life. Continue giving out light in every direction.

Slowly move your attention back to your physical body, to your arms, legs, back, belly, and head. When you are ready, shift over to one side and come to a seated position. Gently open the eyes and sense the light that naturally radiates from your being. Know that you carry this light wherever you go.

Practice Off the Mat

Make a fresh start every morning. Upon waking, sit up in bed, open the curtains or blinds, and, if weather allows, the window. While breathing out, imagine all your negative energies (mistakes, misunderstandings, and fears) leaving your body with the breath. Visualize this energy as black smoke, permeating out into space until it disappears completely. Then, while breathing in, imagine that all the positive energy of the universe (love, joy, compassion, forgiveness) is embracing your body with the breath. Visualize this energy as pure-white light that enters from the pores, eventually pervading every cell within.

Wise Words

When you're connected to spirit, life flows effortlessly, and you perceive the world as a supportive, enjoyable place.

Practicing inner-light visualization meditation will enhance your spiritual development.

The more you practice feeling your own light, the more adept you get at sensing the light in others.

Favorite Place

Intention

To develop the mental ability to go to a place of peace and tranquility whenever the need arises.

Approximate Time

10 minutes

Lesson

Lie in shavasana. Using our imaginations, we will explore our favorite places. Your favorite place could be imaginary or a place you've been. It may be inside or outside, your home, a vacation spot such as a beach or cabin, or it could be a setting of fun and fantasy.

Close your eyes. Take several slow, deep breaths, exhaling completely after each.

Now imagine a location where you feel completely comfortable, peaceful, and safe. It might be real or hypothetical, a place from your past or somewhere you've always wanted to visit. Make it exactly as you want it to be, the right temperature, the right sounds. Are you alone or is someone with you?

Take your time, and allow this special place to take shape slowly. As your place begins to take shape, look around. Look to your left, to your right, and all around you. What do you see? Notice the colors, the textures, the shapes.

Listen to the sounds of your special place. Do you hear waves, birds, music? Maybe it's silent.

Take a deep breath and notice all the smells around you. Perhaps you smell a pine forest, the ocean, or your favorite food.

What do you feel on your skin? A breeze, raindrops, heat, the warm sun on your cheeks?

Now imagine yourself taking a walk through your place. You spot an object on the ground and pick it up. What is it? Is it smooth or rough, natural or man-made? Why have you found this? What does it mean to you?

Relax and enjoy the peace, comfort, and safety of your special place where nothing can harm you. You feel whole and complete. Relax, feeling thankful and happy to be here at this moment. Everything is right, just as it should be.

When you are ready to return to your body, to this physical room, take a deep breath, exhale fully, and turn to one side. At your own pace, come to seated position.

As you sit, envision your special place, your feelings there, and the object you found. Know that your mind is the most powerful tool you have and that you can be in your favorite place whenever you need to destress, reorganize your thoughts, or simply take a five-minute vacation.

Practice Off the Mat

Check in with your environment. Where you spend time has a deep-seated influence over your state of mind. We may not be always aware of this; notice that it is easier to relax and to be at peace in some rooms than in others. Look at the room or space where you practice. Piles of clutter act as constant reminders of things you need to do, and they work counter to your effort to stay grounded in your present practice.

Strong leaders are referred to as visionaries. They can visualize potential as well as flaws. They often plan every detail in their minds before acting.

Powerful imagery crosses many disciplines. The most effective images are the ones that have meaning to you. In health issues, imagine that healthy cells are plump, juicy, and active, while diseased cells are shrinking until they evaporate entirely.

Wise Words

Your imaginary place can be anywhere, at anytime of your life. Close your eyes and relive a favorite childhood memory, or where you were when you found out that you received a promotion, or imagine yourself in the perfect vacation spot.

Imagery can relieve pain, speed healing, and help the body conquer hundreds of ailments, including depression, impotence, and asthma.

Visualization is the brain's method of communicating to our other organs.

Dark Cloud

Intention

To release the dark cloud surrounding our consciousness.

Approximate Time

8 to 10 minutes

Lesson

[Lesson may be practiced while sitting after a reclining relaxation exercise.] We will now experience the practice of Tonglen, a way of connecting with the suffering of the world and of dissolving it in the form of compassion. Bring your awareness into your open heart center to awaken the wisdom and love within. In the space around you, you may want to call on the presence of a divine being. Visualize that this being is sending rays of compassion and wisdom into you.

Imagine that someone in your life who is suffering is sitting with you. Open yourself to this person's suffering, feeling yourself with him or her. Sense a strong intention inside you to release the person from his or her difficulties.

Breathe in the other person's suffering in the form of a dark cloud and visualize it coming into your heart center. As you breathe out, send brilliant light, as well as your healing love, warmth, energy, and compassion to the other person. Breathe in a feeling of hot, dark, and heavy, and breathe out a feeling of cool, bright, and light. Breathe through all the pores of your body.

Continue this breathing gift as long as you wish. At the end of the practice, visualize that your intentions of love and compassion have eliminated that person's suffering entirely. See that person now glowing with peace, joy, and love.

Now imagine others who may also be suffering—friends, coworkers, relatives. Practice taking in their pain and sending back brilliant light, healing love, clarity, and understanding. While doing the practice, feel that all of their negativity has been purified. You now discover a sense of joy that you have been able to free others from their pain. Now dedicate the positive powers of your intentions to everyone in your personal universe, including yourself.

Practice Off the Mat

Morning practice. Rejoice that you are still alive, that you didn't die during the night, and that you are here again today to enjoy another opportunity to achieve something in life.

Repeat a Tonglen affirmation: "May I give my happiness to all beings."

Know that you are not alone. If you find that you have difficulty with self-compassion, visualize that with each in-breath, you are taking in and transforming the suffering of others who are presently experiencing the same kind of loss, sadness, illness, or emotional anguish as you. This will help you accept your own circumstances with more awareness and compassion.

Wise Words

In your personal healing process, it's advantageous to extend genuine acceptance and compassion toward your suffering and fears.

The term *suffering* is sometimes translated as the Sanskrit term *dukkha*. Dukkha also implies that circumstances come together, change, and disappear.

Journey Through the Chakras

Intention

To cleanse and balance the seven major energy centers.

Approximate Time

15 minutes

Lesson

Please lie in shavasana. Take a moment to ground yourself here in this moment, in this body. Follow the breath as it enters your nose and fills your lungs. Breathe from the abdomen, completely filling on the in-breath and emptying your lungs on the out-breath.

Now feel each of your chakras spinning through your spine, from the tip of your pelvis to the crown of your head. As you breathe in, imagine that you are breathing red-earth energy from the soles of your feet, up your legs, and into your root chakra at the tip of the spine. With each new breath, allow more red energy to move up your legs, filling and balancing your root chakra, the center of survival. Imagine the whole room glowing red; feel its strength and power. You can sense this as tingling as the energy fills your root, legs, and feet.

With your next breath, move your awareness up to your second chakra, the center of pleasure. Permit the red-earth energy from your root to move up into the orange energy in your second chakra, at the pelvic center. Take a moment to observe this area. Feel the space around you begin to glow orange. With a tingling sensation, the spirit begins to swirl into this chakra, charging it with vitality. Watch as your orange chakra grows and spins until it extends out from your body.

Now move your awareness up to your third chakra, the center of will and power. Allow the red and orange energy to move up into the yellow energy at the solar plexus. Imagine a golden pulsating glow coming out of your body at the solar plexus, giving you strength, will, and the power to achieve your goals. Feel its rays streaming through each part of your body, filling and warming you.

On your next breath, move your awareness up to your fourth chakra, the heart center. Allow the red, orange, and yellow to move up into the emerald-green energy at the center of your chest, in your spiritual heart. The heart is your connection between the physical and the spiritual states of consciousness. This chakra is the ruler of love, compassion, and wisdom. Release any tensions, imperfections, or impurities. Open your heart with compassion to the world, to all beings. Feel the glowing emerald-green heart intensity from deep within and all around you.

Move your awareness up to your throat center, the fifth chakra, the center of communication. Allow the red, orange, yellow, and green vibrations to move up into the electric-blue energy in your throat. With each new breath, feel the red-earth energy move up your legs, then see it turn orange, yellow, and green. Then let the blue rays extend all around your throat, communicating with all that is around you. Feel the throat open as you recharge this chakra with your positive intentions.

With your next breath, move your awareness up to the sixth chakra, your third eye, your center of intuition. It vibrates to the color indigo and is the house of inner vision and intuition. Allow the red, orange, yellow, green, and blue vibrations to move up into the deep-blue-indigo pulse at the eyebrow center. See the purity of your thoughts as you wash away any toxic images, cleansing and soothing your inner view. Psychic energy is available to you beyond what you may think. Feel the third eye open, indigo streaming from the place between your eyebrows, and note any mental visions as this occurs.

With your next breath, move your awareness up to your crown center, the seventh chakra, and your connection to the divine. Watch the red, orange, yellow, green, blue, and indigo vibrations move up into the vibrant, violet energy in your crown. Reflect on your spirituality and feel the chakra's brilliant-violet presence. Enjoy the violet flowing in as it surrounds your body.

Now see a golden-white aura that extends up and out from the crown chakra and envelopes your whole body. You are completely refreshed, calm, and peaceful. You are balanced on all levels of your consciousness, full of vitality and filled with life force.

Practice Off the Mat

Food for the chakras. Feed yourself in order to help support and fuel your chakras. Whenever one or more of your chakras is unbalanced, you may be overindulging or leaving out foods that nourish that specific chakra.

- Root (survival): Root vegetables, proteins, and spices such as horseradish, hot paprika, chives, and cayenne pepper.
- Sacral (pleasure): Sweet fruits such as melons, mangos, strawberries, passion fruit, and oranges; honey, almonds, and spices such as cinnamon, vanilla, carob, and sesame seeds.
- Solar (will): Granola and grains, including pastas, breads, cereal, rice, flax seed, and sunflower seeds; dairy, including milk, cheeses, and yogurt; spices, including ginger, chamomile, turmeric, cumin, and fennel.
- Heart (love): Leafy vegetables such as spinach, kale, dandelion greens, broccoli, cauliflower, and cabbage, celery, squash; spices such as basil, sage, thyme, cilantro, and parsley.
- Throat (communication): Liquids such as water, fruit juices, herbal teas; lemons, limes, grapefruit, kiwi; spices such as salt, lemon grass, peppermint, and spearmint.
- Brow (intuition): Dark-colored fruits such as blueberries, red grapes, black-berries, raspberries, grape juice, pomegranate juice; spices such as lavender and poppy seed.
- Crown (connection to divine): For inhaling only, not to eat; burn incense and smudge herbs such as sage, copal, myrrh, frankincense, and juniper.

Wise Words

To heal is to bring the chakras into alignment and balance.

Be guided by what intuitively feels right, rather than by what a book or guru or teaching says. This right feeling will continue to evolve as you do. Be your own guru and practice svadhyaya (self-study).

Silent Chanting

Intention

To silently purify the emotions.

Approximate Length

5 to 6 minutes with chanting practice

Lesson

During the course of our busy days, it's tempting to fall mindlessly into noisy distractions that take us away from our true selves. Many of us find that we need to fill the gaps of silence with the noise of radio, television, and talk. We've become afraid of silence, like children afraid of the dark.

When we absorb our mind in chant—the sound that's produced by the body when it is in union with the mind—we experience a purification of the mind. Chant develops our concentration and strength of mind, and it purifies negative emotions. The intentional sound of chant, unlike the noisy fillers of life, enhances the silence around us, balances our inner and outer worlds, and takes us back to our true selves.

The practice of chanting can integrate silence with chant. This is referred to as *silent chanting.* As a result, chanting can be practiced anywhere at anytime.

Applying a three-part exhale, we can silently repeat the three seed syllables found in **aum** in unison with our breathing: *oh* is the seed sound of divine body, *ah* is the seed sound of divine speech, and *mm* is the seed sound of divine thought.

To practice silent chant, exhale the first third of your breath from the third eye to the heart center and mentally say *oh*. Exhale the second third of your breath from heart to navel and mentally say *ah*. Finally, exhale the last third of your breath from navel to public bone and mentally say *mm*, allowing the *mmmm* vibration to continue silently until the last bit of exhale is released. Follow this long exhale with an equally long, silent *om*, inhaling from public bone to the crown.

Feel how the breath connects with the individual and divine body, speech, and mind. Think of these syllables as the universal embodiment of strength, openness, and oneness.

Finally, allow your silent chanting to dissolve into relaxed breathing.

Practice Off the Mat

Sufficiently unaware of his speech, Tom had a habit of making sarcastic and acerbic comments. His words were often interpreted as biting and hurtful. When a friend brought this to his attention, he began to practice the art of thinking before speaking. If you are pushed by a habit to say something unkind, don't say it. Instead, take a notebook and write it down.

Silent chant can be an enlightening tool for affirmation. Use any words that speak to you. For example, if you want to change an attitude or unhealthy element of your lifestyle, thinking *I can do anything* can alter your thinking and provide you with the inner confidence to make the change.

Wise Words

In the silence, you can hear the voice of reason, your inner self, and the divine.

In time you can become master of your words and thought; you know what to say and what not to say.

Words have the power to both destroy and heal.
When words are both true and kind,
they can change our world.

—Buddha

Namaste.

Glossary

adho mukha shvanasana (AH-doh MOO-kah shvah-NAH-sah-nah)—Downward-facing dog pose.

agni sara (AHG-nee SAH-rah)—Yogic fire ignited by breathing practices.

ajna (AHJ-nah)—Sixth chakra, located at the eyebrow center.

ahimsa (Ah-HIM-sah)—Nonharming.

anahata (Ohn-ah-HAH-tah)—Fourth chakra, located at the heart center.

anuloma krama (Ahn-ah-LOH-mah KRAH-mah)—Segmented inhalation.

aparigraha (Ah-PAH-ree-GRAH-hah)—Nonpossessiveness.

ardha baddha padma paschimottanasana (AHR-dah BAH-dah PAHD-mah Pash-ee-moh-tah-NAH-sah-nah)—Half-bound lotus posterior stretch.

ardha chandrasana (AHR-dah Shahn-DRAH-sah-nah)—Half-moon pose.

asana (AH-sah-nah)—Postures or yoga poses; third limb of Raja yoga.

asteya (Ah-STAY-ah)—Nonstealing.

asvini mudra (AHS-vee-nee MOO-drah)—Horse mudra.

ashtanga (AHSH-tahn-gah)—The eight limbs of yoga as described by Patanjali.

avidya (Ah-VEED-yah)—Spiritual tunnel vision; ignorance.

baddha konasana (BAH-dah Koh-NAH-sah-nah)—Bound angle or butterfly pose.

bharadvajasana (Bah-ROD-vah-jah-sah-nah)—Half-lotus twist.

bhujangasana (BOOJ-ahn-GAH-sah-nah)—Cobra pose.

chakra (Shah-KRAH)—Spinning vortex of subtle energy.

chakrasana (Shah-KRAH-sah-nah)—Wheel pose.

chandra namaskara (Shan-drah Nah-mahs-KAH-rah)—Moon salutation.

chaturanga (Chaht-uh-RAHN-gah)—Stick or four-limbs pose.

dhanurasana (Dohn-your-AH-sah-nah)—Bow pose.

dharana (Dah-RAH-nah)—Concentration; the sixth limb of Raja yoga.

dhyana (Dee-YAH-nah)—Meditation; the seventh limb of Raja yoga.

drishti (DRISH-tee)—Focus point.

dukha (DOO-kah)—Suffering.

garudasana (Gah-roo-DAH-sah-nah)—Eagle pose.

gomukhasana (Goh-moo-KHA-sah-nah)—Cow's-face pose.

halasana (Hah-LAH-sah-nah)—Plow pose.

ham (Hum)—Seed sound of the fifth chakra.

hanumanasana (Hah-new-mahn-AHS-ana)—Splits pose.

hatha yoga (HAH-tah YOH-gah)—The physical practice of balancing the solar and lunar currents of human consciousness, representing the dual nature of man.

ida (EE-dah)—The main energy channel that ends in the left nostril, embodying the moon, and connecting to right-brain activity.

ishvara pranidhana (ISH-var-ah PRAH-nee-DAH-nah)—Surrender to divine consciousness.

janu shirshasana (JAH-noo Shur-SHAH-sah-nah)—Head-to-knee pose.

jathara parivartanasana (Jah-TAH-rah Pah-ree-var-TAHN-ah-sah-nah)—Reclining leg lifts with twist.

kapalabhati (Kah-pah-lah-BHA-tee)—Shining-skull breath using controlled but forceful exhalations.

kapotasana (Kah-POH-tah-sah-nah)—Pigeon pose.

kundalini (KOON-dah-lee-nee)—Dormant energy at the base of the spine, awakened through various yoga practices.

kurmasana (Koohr-MAH-sah-nah)—Tortoise pose.

lam (Lum)—Seed sound of the first chakra.

makarasana (MAHK-ah-RAH-sah-nah)—Crocodile pose.

manipura (Mahn-ah-PUR-ah)—Third chakra, located at the solar plexus.

mantra (MAHN-trah)—Sacred sound used in meditation.

marichyasana (MAH-rih-si-AH-sah-nah)—Seated twist.

matsyasana (Mahtz-YAH-sah-nah)—Fish pose.

mula bandha (MOO-lah BAHN-dah)—Root lock.

muladhara (MOO-lah-hah-rah)—Root chakra, located at the perineum.

nadi (NAH-dee)—Subtle energy channel.

nadi shodhana (NAH-dee Shoh-DAH-nah)—Alternate-nostril breathing.

namaste (Nah-MAH stay)—The light in me bows to the light in you.

natarajasana (Nah-tah-raj-AH-sah-nah)—King-dancer pose.

naukasana (Now-KAH-sah-nah)—Reclining boat pose.

navasana (Nah-VAH-sah-nah)—Sitting boat-balance pose.

niyamas (Nee-YAH-mahs)—Observances; the second limb of Raja yoga.

om (Ohm)—Divine sound of the universe.

padmasana (PAHD-mah-sah-nah)—Lotus pose.

parivrtta janu shirshasana (Par-ee-vrit-ah JAH-noo Shur-SHAH-sah-nah)—Revolved head-to-knee pose.

parivrtta trikonasana (Par-ee-vrit-ah Trik-cohn-AH-sah-nah)—Revolved triangle pose.

parivrtta utkatasana (Par-ee-vrit-ah OOT-kah-sah-nah)—Twisting chair pose.

parshvakonasana (Par-shvah-KOH-nah-sah-nah)—Triangle II pose or side angle pose.

parshvottanasana (Par-shvot-TAH-nah-sah-nah)—Angle or pyramid pose.

paschimottanasana (POSH-ee-moh-tah-NAH-sah-nah)—Posterior stretch pose.

Patanjali (Pah-TAHN-joh-lee)—Hindu sage and author of the *Yoga Sutras*.

pingala (Peen-GAH-lah)—The main energy channel that ends in the right nostril, embodies the sun, and is connected to left-brain activity.

prana (PRAH-nah)—Universal energy that animates all living things.

pranayama (PRAH-nah-YAH-mah)—Control of life force; also referred to as breathing exercises; fourth limb of Raja yoga.

prasarita padottanasana (Prah-sa-REE-tah Pah-doh-tahn-AH-sah-nah)—Standing spread-leg forward bend.

pratyahara (PRAH-tyah-HAH-rah)—Withdrawal of the senses; fifth limb of Raja yoga.

Raja yoga (RHA-jah YO-gah)—The Royal Path; eight-limbed path of yoga.

ram (Rum)—Seed sound of the third chakra.

sahasrara (Sah-haz-RAH-rah)—Seventh chakra, located at the crown of the head.

samadhi (Sah-MAH-dee)—The superconscious state, a state of bliss; the eighth limb of Raja yoga.

santosha (San-TOH-shah)—Contentment.

sarvanga padmasana (SAHR-vahn-GAH PAHD-mah-sah-nah)—Lotus shoulderstand.

sarvangasana (SAHR-vahn-GAH-sah-nah)—Shoulderstand.

saucha (Soh-shah)—Purity.

satya (SAHT-yah)—Truth.

setu bandha sarvangasana (SAY-too BAHN-dah SAHR-vahn-GAH-sah-nah)—Bridge pose.

shalabhasana (Shah-lah-BAH-sah-nah)—Locust pose.

shanti (SHAHN-tee)—Peace.

shavasana (Shah-VAH-sah-nah)—Corpse pose.

simhasana (Sim-HAH-sah-nah)—Lion pose.

shirshasana (Sher-SHAH-sah-nah)—Headstand.

sukhasana (Soo-KAH-sah-nah)—Easy pose.

supta sukhasana (Soop-TAH Soo-KAH-sah-nah)—Reclining easy pose.

surya namaskara (SOOR-yah Nah-mahs-KAH-rah)—Sun salutation.

sushumna (Soo-SHOOM-nah)—The central and main nadi that runs along the spine and ends at the crown chakra.

svadhisthana (SVAHD-hiss-tahn-ah)—Second chakra, located at the lower abdomen.

svadhyaya (Svahd-YAH-yah)—Self-study.

tadasana (Ta-DAH-sah-nah)—Mountain pose.

tapas (TAH-pahs)—Determined effort.

tittibhasana (Tee-tah-BAH-sah-nah)—Firefly pose.

trikonasana (Trik-cohn-AH-sah-nah)—Triangle pose.

uddiyana bandha (OO-DEE-anna BAHN-dah)—An energy lock that includes a forceful exhalation followed by a sharp sucking up of the intestines and diaphragm into a vacuum created in the thoracic cavity.

ujjayi (OO-JAH-yee)—A breathing practice that uses an audible vibration by gently closing the glottis in the throat.

upavistha konasana (Oo-pah-VEESH-tah Kohn-NAH-sah-nah)—Seated angle pose.

urdhva mukha shvanasana (OORD-vah MOOK-hah Shvah-NAH-sah-nah)—Upward-facing dog pose.

ustrasana (Oohs-TRAH-sah-nah)—Camel pose.

uttanasana (OOH-tah-NAH-sah-nah)—Standing forward bend.

vam (Vum)—Seed sound of the second chakra.

vasisthasana (Vah-shish-TAHS-ah-nah)—Side plank pose.

vinyasa (Vin-YAH-sah)—A series of asanas that link movement with breath.

virabhadrasana (Veer-ah-bah-DRAH-sah-nah)—Warrior pose.

virasana (Vir-AH-sah-nah)—Hero pose.

visuddha (Vah-SHOE-dah)—Fifth chakra, located at the throat center.

vrikshasana (Vrik-SHAH-sah-nah)—Tree pose.

vrittis (Vrit-EEZ)—Fluctuations of the mind.

yamas (YAH-mahs)—Five restraints; first limb of Raja yoga.

yoga (YOH-gah)—To join or yoke.

Yoga Sutras (YOH-gah SOOT-rahs)—A series of aphorisms relating to the practice of yoga as codified by Patanjali.

Recommended Reading List

This list is merely a drop in the literary ocean of yoga knowledge and guidance. These books just happen to be some of my favorites.

Anderson, Sandra and Solvik, Rolf. *Yoga: Mastering the Basics*. Honesdale, PA: Himalayan Institute Press, 2000.

Anodea, Judith. *Wheels of Life*. St. Paul: Llewellyn, 1998.

Arya, Usharbudh. *Philosophy of Hatha Yoga*. Glenview, IL: Himalayan International Institute of Yoga Science & Philosophy of USA, 1977.

Birch, Beryl Bender. *Beyond Power Yoga*. New York: Fireside, 2000.

Brazier, David. *Zen Therapy: Transcending the Sorrows of the Human Mind*. New York: Wiley, 1996.

Easwaran, Eknath. (Translation) *The Upanishads*. Berkeley, CA: Blue Mountain Center of Meditation, 1987.

Farhi, Donna. *The Breathing Book: Good Health and Vitality Through Essential Breath Work*. New York: Holt, 1996.

Feuerstein, George. *The Shambhala Encyclopedia of Yoga*. Boston: Shambhala, 1997.

Feuerstein, George. (Translation and Commentary) *The Yoga Sutra of Patanjali*. Rochester, VT: Inner Traditions International, 1979, 1989.

Gates, Rolf and Kenison, Katrina. *Meditations From the Mat*. New York: Anchor Books, 2002.

Hanh, Thich Nhat. *Old Path White Clouds*. Berkeley, CA: Parallax Press, 1991.

Iyengar, B.K.S. *Light on Pranayama*. New York: Crossroad, 1998.

Iyengar, B.K.S. *Light on Yoga*. New York: Schocken Books, 1979.

Iyengar, B.K.S. *Yoga: The Path to Holistic Health*. Great Britain: Dorling Kindersley, 2001.

Johnsen, Linda. *Meditation Is Boring: Putting Life In Your Spiritual Practice*. Honesdale, PA: Himalayan Institute Press, 2000.

Kabat-Zinn, John. *Full Catastrophe Living*. New York: Dell, 1990.

Kraftsow, Gary. *Yoga for Wellness*. New York: Penguin, 1999.

Lasater, Judith. *Living Your Yoga: Finding the Spiritual in Everyday Life*. Berkeley, CA: Rodmell Press, 2000.

Lowndes, Florin. *Enlivening the Chakra of the Heart*. Great Britain: Sophia Books, 1998.

Mehta, Silva, Mehta, Mira, and Mehta, Shyam. *Yoga: The Iyengar Way*. New York: Knopf, 1997.

Myss, Caroline. *Anatomy of the Spirit*. New York: Harmony Books, 1996.

Osho. *Meditation: The First and Last Freedom*. New York: St. Martin's Griffin, 1996, 1999.

Prabhavananda, Swami and Isherwood, Christopher. (Translation) *Bhagavad Gita: The Song of God*. Hollywood, CA: Vedanta Press, 1987.

Rama, Swami. *Living With the Himalayan Masters*. Honesdale, PA: Himalayan Institute Press, 1979, 1999.

Rama, Swami. *Meditation and Its Practice*. Honesdale, PA: Himalayan International Institute of Yoga Science & Philosophy, 1992.

Rama, Swami. *Path of Fire and Light*. Honesdale, PA: Himalayan International Institute of Yoga Science & Philosophy, 1986.

Rama, Swami, Ballentine, Rudolph, and Hymes, Alan. *Science of Breath*. Honesdale, PA: Himalayan Institute of Yoga Science & Philosophy, 1979.

Schaeffer, Rachel. *Yoga For Your Spiritual Muscles*. Wheaton, IL: Quest Books, 1998.

Schatz, Mary Pulling. *Back Care Basics*. Berkeley, CA: Rodmell Press, 1992.

Schiffman, Erich. *Yoga: The Spirit and Practice of Moving Into Stillness*. New York: Pocket Books, 1996.

Shunryu, Suzuki. *Zen Mind, Beginner's Mind*. New York: Beacon Press, 1996.

Thondup, Tulku. *The Healing Power of Mind*. Boston, Massachusetts: Shambhala, 1996.

Tigunait, Pandit Rajmani. *At the Eleventh Hour*. Honesdale, PA: Himalayan Institute Press, 2001.

Tigunait, Pandit Rajmani. *The Power of Mantra and The Mystery of Initiation*. Honesdale, PA: Yoga International Books, 1996.

Vishnu-Devananda, Swami. *The Complete Illustrated Book of Yoga*. New York: Harmony Books, 1988.

Vishnu-Devananda, Swami. (Commentary) *Hatha Yoga Pradipika*. New York: OM Lotus, 1987.

Yogananda, Paramahanda. *Autobiography of a Yogi*. Los Angeles: Self-realization fellowship, 1998.

Asana Index

Asana Index   231

About the Author

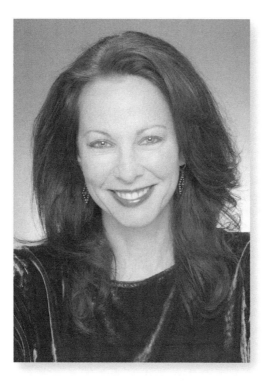

Nancy Gerstein has been a student of yoga for almost 30 years and is a certified hatha yoga teacher with the Himalayan Institute of Yoga Philosophy and Science. Ms. Gerstein is also a reiki master practitioner and yoga therapist.

As a workshop speaker and frequent contributor to *Yoga Chicago Magazine*, Gerstein shares her experience as a yoga teacher and student emphasizing the systematic integration of yogic philosophy into daily living, encouraging her students to take their yoga out of the classroom. She is a member of the Himalayan Institute Teachers Association (HITA), the International Association of Yoga Therapists, Midwest Yoga Teacher's Network, and Yoga Alliance.

Ms. Gerstein resides in Morton Grove, Illinois. In her free time she enjoys hiking and traveling.

For information on Ms. Gerstein's classes and workshops, visit www.guidingyogaslight.com or e-mail her at nancy@guidingyogaslight.com.

About the Model

Howard Davis lives in Los Angeles and has more than 15 years of experience teaching hatha, ashtanga, and kundalini yoga to students of all ages. A graduate of Cambridge University and UCLA, he is the director of Tenth Gate Yoga, which works with corporations and individuals to develop long-term, personalized stress-reduction programs. Employing a variety of healing modalities, including reflexology and gong therapy, he continues to develop his personal sadhana under the instruction of Erich Schiffman at Exhale, Guru Prem Singh Khalsa at Yoga West, and Abbot Tenshin Fletcher at the Zen Mountain Center, near Idyllwild, California. For more information, visit www.tenthgateyoga.com.

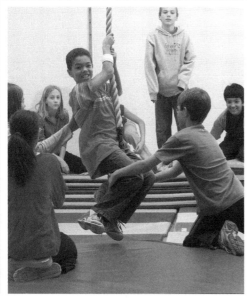
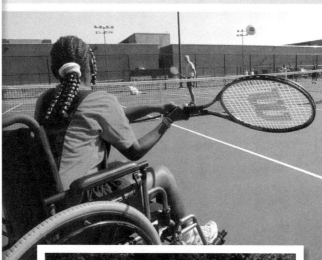
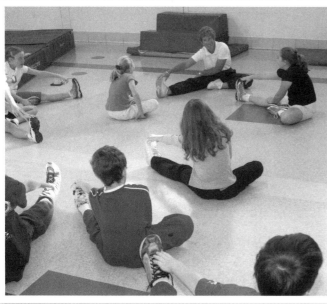
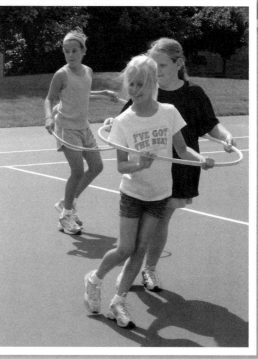
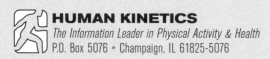